This book is dedicated to my wonderful husband, Donald, for whom I am eternally grateful. His boundless good cheer and support enable me to accomplish my professional and personal goals.

Contributors

Editor

Joyce P. Griffin-Sobel, RN, PhD, AOCN®, APRN,BC
Director of Undergraduate Programs, Associate Professor
Hunter-Bellevue School of Nursing
New York, New York
Editor, *Clinical Journal of Oncology Nursing*
Pittsburgh, Pennsylvania
Chapter 1. Overview of Gastrointestinal Cancers;
Chapter 2. Anatomy and Physiology of the Gastrointestinal Tract;
Chapter 3. Biology, Prevention, and Screening; Chapter 5. Colorectal and Anal Cancers;
Chapter 6. Nursing Care of Patients With Gastrointestinal Cancers;
Chapter 8. Evidence-Based Practice: Where We Are Now

Authors

John S. Macdonald, MD
Medical Director
St. Vincent's Comprehensive Cancer Center
New York, New York
Chief Medical Officer
Aptium Oncology, Inc.
Los Angeles, California
Chapter 4. Esophageal and Gastric Cancers

Denise G. O'Dea, RN, NP, BC, OCN®
Nurse Practitioner
St. Vincent's Comprehensive Cancer Center
New York, New York
Chapter 4. Esophageal and Gastric Cancers

Loleta Samuel-O'Garro, MSN, RN, APRN,BC, AOCN®
Nurse Practitioner
The Cancer Institute of New Jersey
New Brunswick, New Jersey
Chapter 7. Symptom Management of Gastrointestinal
*   Cancers*

Sherri Henry Suozzo, MSN, APN-C, AOCN®
Instructor of Nursing
Seton Hall University
South Orange, New Jersey
Clinical Nurse Specialist, Oncology
Somerset Medical Center
Somerville, New Jersey
Chapter 7. Symptom Management of Gastrointestinal
*   Cancers*

Contents

Preface

Advances in molecular biology, oncology, genetics, and surgical techniques have greatly increased the therapeutic options available to patients with gastrointestinal (GI) cancers and people who are at risk. Research findings on chemoprevention and the role of nutrition in prevention of cancer are equally exciting. However, significant disparities exist in cancer care, despite increasing attention to the issue over recent years.

This book was written for the nurse caring for patients with GI cancer, for excellent nursing care is the constant in guiding patients through their illness. The emphasis in every chapter is on what the nurse needs to know to have an impact on the prevention, treatment, and management of GI cancers. As treatments improve and patients are cured or live longer between therapies, survivorship issues have become increasingly important for the nurse to understand. The reader should become involved in research and education to reduce the health disparities that exist in the United States and to increase the public's awareness of effective preventive strategies against GI cancer. If nurses engage in dialogue with oncology colleagues and public healthcare professionals, real outcomes can be achieved in reducing death rates from many of these preventable cancers.

CHAPTER 1

Overview of Gastrointestinal Cancers

Joyce P. Griffin-Sobel, RN, PhD, AOCN®, APRN,BC

Introduction

Cancers of the gastrointestinal (GI) tract include those of the esophagus, stomach, colon, rectum, and anus. Risk factors, incidence, prevalence, and prognosis vary for each site. Many of the risk factors are modifiable, and in a significant number of cases, the cancers are preventable with proper screening and curable when detected and treated at an early stage.

Esophageal cancer is a treatable but rarely curable cancer. Incidence has increased over the past 20 years in the United States, particularly adenocarcinomas of the esophagus, which have increased by 450% in Caucasian men and 50% in African American men (Enzinger & Mayer, 2003). Squamous cell carcinomas are more common in the rest of the world. Treatment involves surgical resection, whenever possible, followed by chemotherapy and radiotherapy. Men and African Americans have a higher incidence of esophageal cancer than do other groups (Posner, Forastiere, & Minsky, 2005).

Gastric cancer ranks second in cancer deaths across the world. In the United States, incidence has been decreasing dramatically and currently occupies 14th place among cancer incidences (American Cancer Society [ACS], 2006). Adeno-carcinomas represent 90%–95% of all gastric malignancies. Over the past 25 years, the number of gastric cancers occuring at the gastroesophageal (GE) junction and in the cardia has dramatically increased. Treatment for gastric cancer is surgery, followed by chemotherapy and radiotherapy (Pisters, Kelsen, Powell, & Tepper, 2005).

Colorectal cancer (CRC), a preventable, highly treatable, and often curable cancer, is common in men and women. Surgery is the primary form of treatment and results in cure in more than 50% of the patients. Local or distant recurrences develop in many patients after surgical resection, and those with the highest risk of recurrence receive chemotherapy. More than half of the patients are diagnosed at stage III or with metastatic disease, and minorities are diagnosed more often at advanced stages of cancer than Caucasians (Xiong & Ajani, 2004). For the four major cancer sites (prostate, female breast, lung, and CRC), minority populations have a greater risk of cancer death than other groups (Clegg, Li, Hankey, Chu, & Edwards, 2002).

Anal cancers are uncommon, representing 4% of all cancers (Ryan, Compton, & Mayer, 2000). In the United States, squamous cell carcinomas are the most common histology. The risk of developing anal cancers is rising, with people engaging in receptive anal intercourse and with those having a higher number of lifetime sexual partners being at higher risk (Cummings, Ajani, & Swallow, 2005). A strong correlation exists between human papillomavirus (HPV) infection and anal cancer. Treatment consists of surgery, radiation, and chemotherapy (Cummings et al.).

Incidence and Demographics

CRC is the third most common type of cancer in men and women, with an estimated 106,680 cases of colon and 41,930 cases of rectal cancer expected to occur in 2006 (ACS, 2006). Incidence and mortality rates are greatest in developed Western nations (Van Cutsem & Costa, 2005; Wilkes, 2005). Peak incidence is in individuals older than 60, with more women than men developing colon cancer and more men than women acquiring rectal cancer (Wilkes). Seventy percent of patients present with localized disease, and surgery can be curative in these individuals. However, relapses after complete resection are frequent (Van Cutsem & Costa). Polyp removal and fecal occult blood testing reduced the incidence of CRC by 75% and 20%, respectively (Mandel et al., 2000; Winawer et al., 1993).

Individuals residing in high poverty areas are at an increased risk for developing or dying from cancer (Clegg et al., 2002). ACS estimated that more than 16,000 diagnoses of CRC occurred in African Americans in 2005 (Jemal et al., 2005). African Americans have the highest incidence of CRC of any group, and survival rates are lower than for Caucasians (Agrawal et al., 2005). In an analysis of 57,000 patients with rectal cancer entered into the National Cancer Institute (NCI)-funded Surveillance, Epidemiology and End Results (SEER) Cancer Incidence Database, African Americans with rectal cancer were diagnosed at a younger age (mean age 64) than Caucasians (mean age 69) (Morris, Billingsley, Baxter, & Baldwin, 2004). African Americans were diagnosed at a more advanced stage of disease than Caucasians (p < .001); Caucasians were more likely to have sphincter-preserving surgeries than African Americans.

The estimated incidences of other GI cancers in 2006 are 4,660 cases of anal cancer, with 660 deaths; 14,550 new cases of esophageal cancer, with 13,770 deaths; and 22,280 cases of stomach cancer, with 11,430 deaths (Jemal et al., 2006). Esophageal cancer is uncommon in the United States, with a lifetime risk of less than 1%. However, the risk is increasing, along with a shift in histology type and tumor location. Adenocarcinoma is now more prevalent than squamous cell, with a shift to the GE junction and cardia. African American men are more commonly diagnosed with squamous cell carcinomas, and incidence rates in this demographic have substantially decreased from a peak in the 1980s, along with a steady decrease in mortality. Despite this progress, death rates from esophageal cancer in African American men continue to exceed those of all other populations combined. Conversely, incidence in Caucasian men has increased. Esophageal cancer is five times more common in Caucasians than African Americans, and the ratio of male to female incidence is 7:1. Particularly alarming is an increase in the number of adenocarcinomas by more than 400% during the past 20 years; and in Caucasian women, incidence has increased by more than 300%. These changes in incidence are thought to be related to increased rates of both GE reflux and obesity. Survival rates at five years from esophageal cancer are poor, ranging from 5%–30% (Posner et al., 2005).

Gastric cancer has a worldwide incidence of 875,000 new cases annually but is gradually decreasing in many parts of the world because of dietary and food preparation changes. The United States has seen a dramatic decline in gastric cancer to seventh in cancer-related deaths. It continues to be endemic in Japan, Eastern Europe, and South America. It is twice as common in men than in women and 1.5 times more common in African American men than Caucasian men. Mortality has declined in Japan because of mass screening. Death rates are highest for African American men, followed by Caucasian men, African American women, and Caucasian women, in that order. Gastric cancers are being diagnosed more commonly at the proximal stomach and GE junction (Pisters et al., 2005).

Anal cancers are one-tenth as common as rectal cancers, and in North America, 80% are squamous cell carcinomas. Median age at diagnosis is 60–65 years, and it is more common in women. Incidence of the disease is increasing in Caucasian men. Anal cancer is associated with infection by HPV (Ryan et al., 2000). Risk factors include a history of multiple sexual partners in homosexual or heterosexual relationships and receptive anal intercourse. Individuals who are immunosuppressed also are at an increased risk (Cummings et al., 2005).

Race, Ethnicity, and Poverty

NCI (2005) defined health disparities as differences in the incidence, prevalence, mortality, and burden of cancer and related adverse health conditions that exist among specific population groups in the United States. A benchmarking document in cancer health disparities from NCI noted that underserved populations are more likely to be diagnosed and die from preventable cancers, be diagnosed with late-stage disease with cancers for which screening is available for early detection, and receive treatment that does not meet acceptable standards of care (NCI).

African Americans have overall higher cancer incidence and mortality rates compared to other groups. Socioeconomic status may play a large part in these and other disparities, with poverty affecting the likelihood of developing cancer and securing appropriate and timely treatment (NCI, 2005).

CRC is the second most common cancer in African American women and the third most common in African American men (ACS, 2005b). Incidence rates of CRC in African American men and women, while stabilized since 1975, remain higher than in Caucasians (ACS, 2005a). A disproportionate number of cancer deaths occur among racial and ethnic minorities, especially African Americans, who have a 33% higher risk of dying than Caucasians and are twice as likely to die of cancer as Asians and Hispanics (Shavers & Brown, 2002). When looking at cancer among the five major racial and ethnic groups in the United States, African Americans have the highest overall risk of developing cancer, the highest overall risk of dying from cancer, and the poorest indices of cancer survival (Underwood, Powe, Canales, Meade, & Im, 2004). African Americans are diagnosed with CRC at a younger age than Caucasians, which has implications for screening guidelines (Agrawal et al., 2005). More than 7,000 deaths from CRC are expected to occur among African Americans in 2005, and it is the third leading cause of cancer deaths (ACS, 2005a). SEER data from 1998–2002 showed that incidences of CRC in Asian/Pacific Islanders, Native Americans, and Hispanics are lower than that of Caucasians or African Americans (Edwards et al., 2005).

The Institute of Medicine (IOM) documented the disproportionate cancer incidence and death rates in African Americans, regardless of economic and health insurance status, and their lesser chances of receiving the most curative treatments (Smedley, Stite, & Nelson, 2002). The report described a complex interplay among economic, social, and cultural factors. A study of 4,706 patients with CRC showed that Caucasians received standard adjuvant therapy significantly more often than African Americans (Potosky, Harlan, Kaplan, Johnson, &

Lynch, 2002; Shavers & Brown, 2002). Similar findings have been demonstrated in lung cancer (Bach, Cramer, Warren, & Begg, 1999) and in receipt of intensive care in general (Fiscella & Franks, 2000; Fiscella, Franks, Gold, & Clancy, 2000). A comprehensive literature review found limited evidence of differences in treatment effectiveness among racial or ethnic groups but only in receipt of definitive therapies (Shavers & Brown). Freeman (2004) asserted that racial and ethnic bias of healthcare professionals influences the quality of healthcare delivery. Survival rates are lower for African Americans than Caucasians who present with the same disease stage (Potosky et al.). In an equal-access system such as the U.S. Veterans Affairs Health Care System, no survival difference exists between African Americans and Caucasians (Dominitz, Samsa, Landsman, & Provenzale, 1998).

Many African Americans, including older adults and those living in rural and medically underserved communities, do not have ready access to quality cancer care facilities (Underwood et al., 2004). Rural communities, where 14% of African Americans reside, have limited access to quality cancer care; urban communities, with 55% of the African American population, have a shortage of healthcare providers and services. An analysis of doctor visits by Medicare beneficiaries older than 65 years of age found that African Americans were treated by physicians who were less likely to be board certified, and those physicians reported greater difficulties in obtaining specialized care for their patients (Bach, Pham, Schrag, Tate, & Hargraves, 2004). Some authors suggested that African Americans and Hispanics are adequately represented in clinical trials (Hutchins, Unger, Crowley, Coltman, & Albain, 1999), whereas others have noted that racial and ethnic minorities and older adults are less likely to enroll in those trials (Murthy, Krumholz, & Gross, 2004).

In 2002, the U.S. census reported 12% of Americans were poor, 15% were uninsured, and a disproportionate percentage of minorities were poor (Proctor & Dalaker, 2003). Freeman (2004) reported that 20% of African Americans and 32% of Hispanics are uninsured. Poverty is associated with poorer cancer outcomes, regardless of race or ethnic group (Muss, 2001; Wrigley et al., 2003). Five-year survival rates from cancer are 10% lower for those living in poverty (Ward et al., 2004). In a study of 4,675 women with breast cancer, a 49% higher risk of death was found for uninsured people than for those privately insured, and a 40% higher risk of death was reported for Medicaid patients even after adjusting for age, race, income, comorbidities, and stage of disease (Ayanian, Kohler, Abe, & Epstein, 1993).

A group of more than 1,000 patients with CRC was surveyed about their cancer care after nine months of treatment (Ayanian et al., 2005). Those reporting more problems with obtaining health or treatment information, psychosocial care, or coordination of care were more likely to be Asian/Pacific Islander, Hispanic, and African American. Patients who were non-Caucasian and non-English-speaking were less likely to

rate their quality of cancer care as very good or excellent. Problems with coordination of care were most strongly correlated with poor quality-of-care ratings. Because differences exist in cancer treatment and outcomes by race, ethnicity, and language (Smedley et al., 2002), perhaps these interpersonal and communication-related problems may be contributory.

Age

The incidence of all GI cancers, as with many other cancers, increases with age. The U.S. Census Bureau estimated that 12.6% of the population is 65 and older, and this percentage is projected to increase to 20.3%, or 70 million people, by 2030 (Kinsella & Velkoff, 2001). Cancer occurs more frequently and causes more deaths in older adults. Sixty percent of malignancies occur in people older than 65, but they receive adjuvant chemotherapy less often than younger people (Sargent et al., 2001). In a medical review of 4,706 people with CRC, those younger than age 55 received standard therapy 78% of the time, whereas those older than 80 received standard therapy only 24% of the time (Potosky et al., 2002). This sharp decline in the use of standard chemotherapy, beginning at the age of 75, is suggestive of age bias even after adjusting for tumor grade and comorbidities. A growing body of knowledge suggests that chemotherapy can be safe and effective in older adults. For many types of cancer chemotherapy treatment, no difference in toxicities is seen in people older than 70 years (Muss, 2001). A meta-analysis of phase III randomized trials in CRC involving 3,351 patients demonstrated that overall survival from CRC was higher in older adults who received adjuvant therapy than those who were untreated, with no significantly higher incidence of GI symptoms, leukopenia, or stomatitis compared to younger people (Sargent et al.). Other studies supported that older adults tolerate and respond to chemotherapy (Benson et al., 1991; Giovanazzi-Bannon, Rademaker, Lai, & Benson, 1994).

Conversely, some studies have suggested that older adults with cancer may be more susceptible to toxicities such as myelosuppression, GI distress, renal impairment, and cardiotoxicities (Crivellari et al., 2000; Morrison et al., 2001). When compared to younger patients, older adults with cancer develop myelosuppression more frequently and with greater severity (Morrison et al.), are more susceptible to cardiotoxicity (Kimmick, Fleming, Muss, & Balducci, 1997), and are at increased risk for GI distress such as mucositis, nausea, vomiting, and diarrhea. However, it is important to note that some of those studies included few older adults, were reviews of the literature, or were based on anecdotal information.

Older adults are underrepresented in cancer clinical trials (Hutchins et al., 1999). Eligibility criteria of standard clinical trials often exclude many comorbidities, and little is known about the ability of older adults with normal age-related organ impairments to tolerate treatment. Similarly, physicians may not recommend participation in clinical trials because of assumptions about the ability of this population to withstand cancer treatments. Benson et al. (1991) reported that in a survey of American oncologists, 50% decided whether a patient was unsuitable for a clinical trial based on age alone. Family members also believed the trials might be too toxic for older patients (Benson et al.). A retrospective analysis of 55 cancer clinical trials reported a statistically significant underrepresentation of older adults (Talarico, Chen, & Pazdur, 2004). This underrepresentation was found in all cancers except for hormonal treatments for breast cancer and was most predominant for those older than 70 years of age.

Risk Factors

Many risk factors for GI cancers are modifiable, although the most research has been conducted on CRC. Approximately 90% of all instances of CRC and deaths are thought to be preventable through lifestyle changes (Herdman & Lichtenfeld, 2004). Etiologies of CRC have been studied extensively, and diet, physical activity, weight, and smoking have well-documented links to its development. The highly complex interactions between inherited susceptibility and external factors are under active investigation to determine the most effective prevention strategies.

Personal and Familial Risk

Average-risk individuals, with no familial history of cancer or polyps, comprise the majority of those who develop CRC. Intermediate-risk individuals have a personal or familial history of colorectal polyps or CRC, placing them at higher risk for the disease. People with a history of a colon cancer are at an increased risk for a second (metachronous) cancer, in addition to risk for recurrence (Winawer et al., 1996). Patients with a familial risk, those who have two or more first- or second-degree relatives with CRC or adenomatous polyps, represent approximately 20% of all cases of the disease. They have approximately twice the risk of developing CRC as someone without a family history. The risk is higher if more than one first-degree relative is affected (Winawer et al., 1996). High-risk individuals are those with a genetic syndrome, which is discussed later.

Diet

Drawing conclusions from dietary studies is difficult because recall is imperfect, and amounts of food or methods of cooking rarely are included in the database. Additionally, childhood dietary data rarely are included in studies examining dietary effect on CRC incidence, which is a significant limitation to these data (Willett, 2005). However, migrant and other studies have shown that risk for CRC is modifiable and related to lifestyle factors (Miller et al., 1996). Colon cancer

risk changes as people move from low- to high-incidence areas, demonstrating the importance of adult environmental exposure.

Meat and Fat

In several large, well-designed studies, including a meta-analysis and the Nurses' Health Study, high meat consumption was related to the development of CRC (Chao et al., 2005; Norat, Lukanova, Ferrari, & Riboli, 2002; Willett, Stampfer, Colditz, Rosner, & Speizer, 1990). The fatty acid content of red meat may be particularly harmful, and promoters of carcinogenesis may be formed when it is cooked (Giovannucci et al., 1995). No increase in risk with meat consumption was seen in two other large studies (Bostick et al., 1993; Thun et al., 1992). High fat intake increased the risk of adenoma recurrence in one study (Neugut et al., 1993), but another found that a low-fat, high-fiber diet did not affect recurrence rate (Schatzkin et al., 2000). A high dietary glycemic load is associated with an increased risk of CRC (Higginbotham et al., 2004). This effect may be related to a relationship between hyperinsulinemia and insulin resistance and tumor growth. Dietary and lifestyle risk factors for developing insulin resistance, such as physical inactivity, obesity, and positive energy balance, also increase the risk of developing CRC and other cancers (Colditz, Cannuscio, & Frazier, 1997; Giovannucci et al., 1995; Giovannucci, Colditz, Stampfer, & Willett, 1996).

Fruits and Vegetables

Despite common preconceptions, diets high in fiber, fruits, and vegetables have not decreased the rate of adenoma recurrence or overall cancer incidence (Fuchs et al., 1999). The Nurses' Health Study, with a sample size of 71,910 women, and the Health Professionals Follow-Up Study, with a sample size of 37,725, found no association between fruit and vegetable intake and colon or rectal cancer incidence (Hung et al., 2004). Trials incorporating large doses of fruits and vegetables and beta-carotene also failed to decrease cancer incidence and actually suggested a harmful effect (Willett, 2005). Studies looking at dietary fiber, specifically, have yielded mixed results. No association between fiber intake and CRC was found in a number of large studies (Fuchs et al., 1999; Michels et al., 2000). Other studies have found an inverse relationship between dietary fiber and adenomas (Bingham et al., 2003; Peters et al., 2003). In other studies, the protective effect of fruits and vegetables, particularly those eaten raw, has been shown in esophageal cancer (Posner et al., 2005).

Calcium

In some studies, calcium supplementation decreased the risk of all types of polyps, both malignant and benign. Total calcium intake above 1,200 mg is necessary. Subjects with a high intake of total dietary fiber experienced more pronounced effects of calcium supplementation than those with lower fiber intake (Wallace et al., 2004). A higher consumption of calcium products, including dairy, is associated with a lower risk of CRC and polyp recurrences (Baron et al., 1999; Bonithon-Kopp, Kronborg, Giacosa, Rath, & Faivre, 2000; Cho et al., 2004). This inverse association has been consistent across studies and gender. Combinations of calcium and vitamin D may be the preferred preventive regimen. However, a recent report from a randomized trial of more than 36,000 postmenopausal women from the Women's Health Initiative (WHI) demonstrated that daily supplementation of calcium carbonate with vitamin D for seven years had no effect on the incidence of CRC (Wactawski-Wende et al., 2006). Fifty-four percent of the women were taking calcium supplements at the start of the study, which raises questions about the impact of the intervention. Another limitation was that the average length of intervention was 7 years, which is less than the 10–20 years estimated for the development of CRC. Other possible dietary factors that positively influence risk for CRC include multivitamin and folate use (Fuchs et al., 2002; Giovannucci et al., 1998).

Nonsteroidal Anti-Inflammatory Drugs

Use of anti-inflammatory drugs, particularly aspirin, sulindac, and nonsteroidal anti-inflammatory drugs (NSAIDs), is associated with a decreased incidence of CRC (Thun, Namboodiri, Calle, Flanders, & Heath, 1993; Thun, Namboodiri, & Heath, 1991). Studies in chemoprevention in esophageal and gastric cancers suggest a similar preventive effect (Farrow et al., 1998). These drugs have been found to prevent adenoma formation and to cause adenomatous polyps to regress in patients with histories of CRC, polyp formation, and familial adenomatous polyposis (FAP) (NCI, 2005).

Taking aspirin daily for as little as three years was shown to reduce the development of polyps by 19%–35% in people at high risk for CRC in two randomized clinical trials, confirming numerous earlier observational studies suggesting that regular use of aspirin lowered rates of colorectal adenomas (Baron, Cole, & Sandler, 2003; Sandler et al., 2003). In a large study of healthcare professionals, aspirin was associated with a 30% reduction in CRC and a 50% reduction in advanced cases (Giovannucci, Rimm, Stampfer, Colditz, et al., 1994). Among a group of more than 600,000 adults enrolled in an ACS study, mortality in regular users of aspirin was approximately 40% lower for cancers of the colon and rectum (Smalley, Ray, Daugherty, & Griffin, 1999; Thun et al., 1991). Another large study found no decrease in CRC at 5 years and later at 12 years (Gann, Manson, Glynn, Buring, & Hennekens, 1993; Smalley et al.; Sturmer et al., 1998). At present, the minimal effective dose and duration of use of aspirin is not well defined. In the Nurses' Health Study, beneficial effects were not obvious until after two decades of regular aspirin consumption. Risks of treatment include upper GI bleeding, gastric distress, and hemorrhagic stroke (Baron et al., 2003; Sandler et al.).

Cyclooxygenase (COX) has an inflammatory effect biologically. COX-2 is consistently overexpressed in a large percentage and variety of human tumors, including many CRCs. COX inhibitors include indomethacin, sulindac, piroxicam, ibuprofen, and celecoxib. COX-2 inhibitors are being studied as potential agents in the prevention and treatment of cancer after a century of widespread use for inflammation, fever, and pain. COX-2 inhibitors have been shown to reduce the growth of polyps and are being studied for their anticancer effects. The U.S. Food and Drug Administration has approved the use of celecoxib in those with FAP. In a randomized controlled trial of individuals with FAP, the experimental groups who took 800 mg a day of celecoxib had a 30.7% reduction in polyps and had a 14.6% reduction on 200 mg a day (Steinbach et al., 2000).

Inflammatory Bowel Disease

Inflammatory bowel disease is associated with an increased risk of CRC, and risk increases with the duration of the disease (Wilkes, 2005). Individuals with ulcerative colitis have an absolute risk of CRC of 30% 35 years after diagnosis; this risk increases to 40% for those diagnosed with colitis before 15 years of age (Ekbom, Helmick, Zack, & Adami, 1990).

Smoking and Alcohol

Smokers have a significantly elevated risk of adenomas and CRC (Giovannucci & Martinez, 1996; Giovannucci, Rimm, Stampfer, Hunter, et al., 1994; Neugut, Jacobson, & DeVivo, 1993), but the effect is seen after years of exposure. Men who had smoked for more than 30 years had nearly double the risk of colon cancer compared to nonsmokers, as did women who smoked for more than 40 years. A majority of studies support an association between alcohol use and increased risk for CRC and adenoma formation (Herdman & Lichtenfeld, 2004).

Tobacco and alcohol are major contributing factors to the development of esophageal cancer throughout the world. Ninety percent of the risk for squamous cell cancer can be attributed to tobacco and alcohol. Those who quit smoking experience approximately a 50% reduction in the risk of developing squamous cell cancer of the esophagus. Smoking also is a risk factor for the development of adenocarcinoma, but quitting smoking does not decrease the risk for decades. In the United States, 80% of squamous cell carcinomas in men can be attributed to drinking more than one alcoholic beverage per day (Posner et al., 2005).

Hormone Supplementation

In some studies, postmenopausal female hormone supplementation decreased the risk of colon cancer (Calle, Miracle-McMahill, Thun, & Heath, 1995; Terry et al., 2002), but in the WHI data (Chlebowski et al., 2004), women randomized to hormone replacement had fewer invasive CRCs than the placebo group. However, the experimental group had higher percentages of more advanced lesions than the control group.

Obesity and Physical Activity

Obesity is responsible for at least 10% of CRCs and 25%–40% of esophageal, endometrial, and kidney cancers (Gotay, 2005). Obesity is associated with a twofold increase in risk of CRC in women (Terry, Miller, & Rohan, 2002) and a higher incidence and increased mortality from CRC in both genders (Rosen & Schneider, 2004). Exercise, in particular, conferred high levels of protection when vigorous and long-standing (Giovannucci et al., 1996). Physical activity also lowers one's risk of developing large adenomatous polyps, suggesting it may act at an early point in the carcinogenic process. This effect is seen across all weight levels, suggesting a benefit of physical activity for cancer prevention as well as weight loss (Giovannucci et al., 1995, 1996; Herdman & Lichtenfeld, 2004).

Increased body mass index (BMI) is a risk factor for adenocarcinoma of the esophagus, with the highest risk (sevenfold) for those with the highest BMI. Obesity also is thought to contribute to increased risk of gastric cancer (Calle, Rodriguez, Walker-Thurmond, & Thun, 2003).

When a Mediterranean diet is adopted, with an emphasis on fish, nuts, poultry, and legumes, along with other health lifestyle factors, such as regular exercise, approximately 70% of colon cancers can be avoided (Hu & Willett, 2002; Platz et al., 2000).

Health Literacy

A study evaluating patient time and resource use associated with the delivery of chemotherapy and management of neutropenia demonstrated that even relatively simple visits resulted in large disruptions of patient time and lifestyle before, during, and after the visit (Fortner et al., 2004). Cancer treatment is a stressful experience for patients. During the course of diagnosis and treatment, patients experience a myriad of symptoms, psychological reactions, disruptions of normal life, and financial burdens. Research consistently has shown that patients with cancer want information about their disease and treatment, but they continue to report that they are not receiving sufficient information to successfully cope with treatment (Skalla, Bakitas, Furstenberg, Ahles, & Henderson, 2004). Patients with cancer want the maximum amount of information about their illness (Chelf et al., 2001). Benefits of providing patients with information include an increased participation in treatment decision making, enhanced ability to cope with treatment, and increased patient satisfaction. Informational needs change as patients move from diagnosis through treatment, requiring dynamic assessment (Adams, 1991; Mills & Sullivan, 1999).

Although informational needs exist across the continuum of cancer care, multiple factors influence patients' ability to access care and to learn. These factors include health literacy, coping style, emotional state, motivation to learn, anxiety, fatigue, cultural background, and environmental factors (Chelf et al., 2001). To navigate the healthcare system effectively, an individual should have skills to understand appointment slips, oral and written communication, and health insurance forms while actively participating in healthcare decisions and learning self-care techniques. Anyone can feel overwhelmed by the amount of material to assimilate; however, those with limitations in language, health literacy, or recall are particularly at risk. Health literacy, as defined by IOM, is the degree to which individuals have the capacity to obtain, process, and understand basic health information and services needed to make appropriate health decisions (Nielesen-Bohlman, Panzer, & Kindig, 2004).

An IOM report on health literacy stated that one-quarter of the U.S. population is functionally illiterate, another 50 million have marginal literacy skills, and the problem is especially prevalent among older adults (Nielesen-Bohlman et al., 2004). Literacy issues raise concerns about individuals' ability to gain access to and effectively function within the healthcare system. One study reported that one-third to a majority of English-speaking patients, particularly older adults and the chronically ill, at public hospitals could not understand basic health-related materials or instructions about making an appointment and could not comprehend a consent form (Williams et al., 1995). Literacy influences health status and use of health services (Baker, Parker, Williams, & Nurss, 1997; Williams, Baker, Parker, & Nurss, 1998). Literacy was a stronger correlate of health status than education level or sociodemographic variables (Baker et al.).

Summary

Patterns of incidence and prevalence of GI cancers demonstrate the need for improved screening techniques and investigation into root causes of cancer disparities. Modifiable risk factors must be addressed on a societal, individual, and community level. Providing the appropriate amount and type of information also should be a priority. The difficulty with linking diet to cancer incidence or prevention limits prescriptive nutritional recommendations.

References

Adams, M. (1991). Information and education across the phases of cancer care. *Seminars in Oncology Nursing, 7,* 105–111.

Agrawal, S., Bhupinderjit, A., Bhutani, M., Boardman, L., Nguyen, C., Romero, Y., et al. (2005). Colorectal cancer in African Americans. *American Journal of Gastroenterology, 100,* 515–523.

American Cancer Society. (2005a). *Cancer facts and figures for African Americans, 2005–2006.* Atlanta, GA: Author.

American Cancer Society. (2005b). *Colorectal cancer facts and figures, special edition.* Atlanta, GA: Author.

American Cancer Society. (2006). *Cancer facts and figures, 2006.* Atlanta, GA: Author.

Ayanian, J.Z., Kohler, B., Abe, T., & Epstein, A. (1993). The relation between health insurance coverage and clinical outcomes among women with breast cancer. *New England Journal of Medicine, 329,* 326–331.

Ayanian, J.Z., Zaslavsky, A.M., Guadagnoli, E., Fuchs, C.S., Yost, K.J., Creech, C.M., et al. (2005). Patients' perceptions of quality of care for colorectal cancer by race, ethnicity, and language. *Journal of Clinical Oncology, 23,* 6576–6586.

Bach, P.B., Cramer, L.D., Warren, J.L., & Begg, C.B. (1999). Racial differences in the treatment of early-stage lung cancer. *New England Journal of Medicine, 341,* 1198–1205.

Bach, P.B., Pham, H., Schrag, D., Tate, R., & Hargraves, J. (2004). Primary care physicians who treat blacks and whites. *New England Journal of Medicine, 351,* 575–584.

Baker, D., Parker, R., Williams, M., & Nurss, J. (1997). The relationship of patient reading ability to self reported health and use of health services. *American Journal of Public Health, 87,* 1027–1030.

Baron, J.A., Beach, M., Mandel, J.S., van Stolk, R.U., Haile, R.W., Sandler, R.S., et al. (1999). Calcium supplements for the prevention of colorectal adenomas. *New England Journal of Medicine, 340,* 101–107.

Baron, J.A., Cole, B.F., & Sandler, R.S. (2003). Randomized trial of aspirin to prevent colorectal adenomas in patients with previous colorectal cancer. *New England Journal of Medicine, 348,* 891–899.

Benson, A., Pregler, J., Bean, J., Rademaker, A., Eshler, B., & Anderson, K. (1991). Oncologists' reluctance to accrue patients onto clinical trials. *Journal of Clinical Oncology, 9,* 2067–2075.

Bingham, S.A., Day, N.E., Luben, R., Ferrari, P., Slimani, N., Norat, T., et al. (2003). Dietary fibre in food and protection against colorectal cancer in the European prospective investigation into cancer and nutrition (EPIC): An observational study. *Lancet, 361,* 1496–1501.

Bonithon-Kopp, C., Kronborg, O., Giacosa, A., Rath, U., & Faivre, J. (2000). Calcium and fibre supplementation in prevention of colorectal adenoma recurrence: A randomized intervention trial. European Cancer Prevention Organization Study Group. *Lancet, 356,* 1300–1306.

Bostick, R., Potter, J.D., Sellers, T., McKenzie, D.R., Kushi, L.H., & Folsom, A.R. (1993). Relation of calcium, vitamin D, and dairy food intake to incidence of colon cancer among older women. The Iowa Women's Health Study. *American Journal of Epidemiology, 137,* 1302–1317.

Calle, E.E., Miracle-McMahill, H., Thun, M.J., & Heath, C.W., Jr. (1995). Estrogen replacement therapy and risk of fatal colon cancer in a prospective cohort of postmenopausal women. *Journal of the National Cancer Institute, 87,* 517–523.

Calle, E., Rodriguez, C., Walker-Thurmond, K., & Thun, M. (2003). Overweight, obesity and mortality from cancer in a prospectively studied cohort of U.S. adults. *New England Journal of Medicine, 348,* 1625–1638.

Chao, A., Thun, M.J., Connell, C.J., McCullough, M.L., Jacobs, E.J., Flanders, W.D., et al. (2005). Meat consumption and risk of colorectal cancer. *JAMA, 293,* 172–182.

Chelf, J., Agre, P., Axelrod, A., Cheney, L., Cole, D., Conrad, K., et al. (2001). Cancer-related patient education: An overview of the last decade of evaluation and research. *Oncology Nursing Forum, 28,* 1139–1147.

Chlebowski, R., Wactawski-Wende, J., Ritenbaugh, C., Hubbell, F.A., Ascensao, J., Rodabough, R.J., et al. (2004). Estrogen plus progestin and colorectal cancer in postmenopausal women. *New England Journal of Medicine, 350,* 991–1004.

Cho, E., Smith-Warner, S.A., Spiegelman, D., Beeson, W.L., van den Brandt, P.A., Colditz, G.A., et al. (2004). Dairy foods, calcium, and colorectal cancer: A pooled analysis of 10 cohort studies. *Journal of the National Cancer Institute, 96,* 1015–1022.

Clegg, L., Li, F., Hankey, B., Chu, K., & Edwards, B.K. (2002). Cancer survival among U.S. whites and minorities. *Archives of Internal Medicine, 162,* 1985–1993.

Colditz, G.A., Cannuscio, C.C., & Frazier, A.L. (1997). Physical activity and reduced risk of colon cancer: Implications for prevention. *Cancer Causes and Control, 8,* 649–667.

Crivellari, D., Bonetti, M., Castiglione-Gertsch, M., Gelber, R., Rudenstam, C., Thurlimann, B., et al. (2000). Burdens and benefits of adjuvant cyclophosphamide, methotrexate and fluorouracil and tamoxifen for elderly patients with breast cancer: The International Breast Cancer Study Group Trial VII. *Journal of Clinical Oncology, 16,* 1412–1422.

Cummings, B., Ajani, J., & Swallow, C. (2005). Cancer of the anal region. In V.T. DeVita, S. Hellman, & S. Rosenberg (Eds.), *Cancer: Principles and practice of oncology* (7th ed., pp. 1125–1137). Philadelphia: Lippincott Williams & Wilkins.

Dominitz, J., Samsa, G., Landsman, P., & Provenzale, D. (1998). Race, treatment and survival among colorectal carcinoma patients in an equal-access medical system. *Cancer, 82,* 2312–2320.

Edwards, B.K., Brown, M.L., Wingo, P.A., Howe, H.L., Ward, E., Ries, L.A.G., et al. (2005). Annual report to the nation on the status of cancer, 1975–2002, featuring population-based trends in cancer treatment. *Journal of the National Cancer Institute, 97,* 1407–1427.

Ekbom, A., Helmick, C., Zack, M., & Adami, H.O. (1990). Ulcerative colitis and colorectal cancer. A population-based study. *New England Journal of Medicine, 323,* 1228–1233.

Enzinger, P., & Mayer, R. (2003). Esophageal cancer. *New England Journal of Medicine, 349,* 2241–2252.

Farrow, D.C., Vaughan, T.L., Hansten, P.D., Stanford, J.L., Risch, H.A., Gammon, M.D., et al. (1998). Use of aspirin and other nonsteroidal anti-inflammatory drugs and risk of esophageal and gastric cancer. *Cancer Epidemiology, Biomarkers and Prevention, 7,* 97–102.

Fiscella, K., & Franks, P. (2000). Individual income, income inequality, health, and mortality: What are the relationships? *Health Services Research, 35*(1 Pt. 2), 307–318.

Fiscella, K., Franks, P., Gold, M.R., & Clancy, C.M. (2000). Inequality in quality: Addressing socioeconomic, racial, and ethnic disparities in health care. *JAMA, 28,* 2579–2584.

Fortner, B., Okon, T., Zhu, K., Tauer, K., Moore, K., & Templeton, D. (2004, May). *Human resource costs and patient time affected by the delivery of chemotherapy and neutropenia management.* Paper presented at the annual meeting of the American Society of Clinical Oncology, New Orleans, LA.

Freeman, H. (2004). Poverty, culture and social injustice: Determinants of cancer disparities. *CA: A Cancer Journal for Clinicians, 54,* 72–77.

Fuchs, C., Giovannucci, E.L., Colditz, G.A., Hunter, D.J., Stampfer, M.J., Rosner, B., et al. (1999). Dietary fiber and the risk of colorectal cancer and adenoma in women. *New England Journal of Medicine, 340,* 169–176.

Fuchs, C.S., Willett, W.C., Colditz, G.A., Hunter, D.J., Stampfer, M.J., Speizer, F.E., et al. (2002). The influence of folate and multivitamin use on the familial risk of colon cancer in women. *Cancer Epidemiology, Biomarkers and Prevention, 11,* 227–234.

Gann, P., Manson, J., Glynn, R., Buring, J.E., & Hennekens, C.H. (1993). Low-dose aspirin and incidence of colorectal tumors in a randomized trial. *Journal of the National Cancer Institute, 85,* 1220–1224.

Giovanazzi-Bannon, S., Rademaker, A., Lai, G., & Benson, A. (1994). Treatment tolerance of elderly cancer patients entered onto phase II clinical trials. *Journal of Clinical Oncology, 12,* 2447–2452.

Giovannucci, E., Ascherio, A., Rimm, E.B., Colditz, G.A., Stampfer, M.J., & Willett, W.C. (1995). Physical activity, obesity, and risk for colon cancer and adenoma in men. *Annals of Internal Medicine, 122,* 327–334.

Giovannucci, E., Colditz, G.A., Stampfer, M.J., & Willett, W.C. (1996). Physical activity, obesity, and risk of colorectal adenoma in women (United States). *Cancer Causes and Control, 7*(2), 253–263.

Giovannucci, E., & Martinez, M. (1996). Tobacco, colorectal cancer, and adenomas: A review of the evidence. *Journal of the National Cancer Institute, 88,* 1717–1730.

Giovannucci, E., Rimm, E.B., Stampfer, M.J., Colditz, G.A., Ascherio, A., & Willett, W.C. (1994). Aspirin use and the risk for colorectal cancer and adenoma in male health professionals. *Annals of Internal Medicine, 121,* 241–246.

Giovannucci, E., Rimm, E.B., Stampfer, M.J., Hunter, D., Rosner, B.A., Willett, W.C., et al. (1994). A prospective study of cigarette smoking and risk of colorectal adenoma and colorectal cancer in U.S. men. *Journal of the National Cancer Institute, 86,* 183–191.

Giovannucci, E., Stampfer, M.J., Colditz, G.A., Hunter, D.J., Fuchs, C., Rosner, B.A., et al. (1998). Multivitamin use, folate, and colon cancer in women in the Nurses' Health Study. *Annals of Internal Medicine, 129,* 517–524.

Gotay, C. (2005). Behavior and cancer prevention. *Journal of Clinical Oncology, 23,* 301–310.

Herdman, R., & Lichtenfeld, L. (2004). *Fulfilling the potential of cancer prevention and early detection: An American Cancer Society and Institute of Medicine symposium.* Washington, DC: Institute of Medicine.

Higginbotham, S., Zhang, Z.F., Lee, I.M., Cook, N.R., Giovannucci, E., Buring, J.E., et al. (2004). Dietary glycemic load and risk of colorectal cancer in the Women's Health Study. *Journal of the National Cancer Institute, 96,* 229–233.

Hu, F.B., & Willett, W. (2002). Optimal diets for prevention of coronary heart disease. *JAMA, 288,* 2569–2578.

Hung, H.C., Joshipura, K.J., Jiang, R., Hu, F.B., Hunter, D., Smith-Warner, S.A., et al. (2004). Fruit and vegetable intake and risk of major chronic disease. *Journal of the National Cancer Institute, 96,* 1577–1584.

Hutchins, L.F., Unger, J.M., Crowley, J.J., Coltman, C.A., Jr., & Albain, K.S. (1999). Underrepresentation of patients 65 years of age or older in cancer-treatment trials. *New England Journal of Medicine, 341,* 2061–2067.

Jemal, A., Murray, T., Ward, E., Samuels, A., Tiwari, R.C., Ghafoor, A., et al. (2005). Cancer statistics, 2005. *CA: A Cancer Journal for Clinicians, 55,* 10–30.

Jemal, A., Siegel, R., Ward, E., Murray, T., Xu, J., Smigal, C., et al. (2006). Cancer statistics, 2006. *CA: A Cancer Journal for Clinicians, 56,* 106–130.

Kimmick, G., Fleming, T.R., Muss, H., & Balducci, L. (1997). Cancer chemotherapy in older adults. *Drugs and Aging, 10*(1), 34–49.

Kinsella, K., & Velkoff, V. (2001). U.S. Census Bureau P95/01-1: An aging world: 2001. Washington, DC: U.S. Government Printing Office.

Mandel, J., Church, T.R., Bond, J.H., Ederer, F., Geisser, M.S., Mongin, S.J., et al. (2000). The effect of fecal occult blood screening on the incidence of colorectal cancer. *New England Journal of Medicine, 343,* 1603–1607.

Michels, K.B., Edward, G., Joshipura, K.J., Rosner, B.A., Stampfer, M.J., Fuchs, C.S., et al. (2000). Prospective study of fruit and vegetable consumption and incidence of colon and rectal cancers. *Journal of the National Cancer Institute, 92,* 1740–1752.

Miller, B., Kolonel, L., Bernstein, L., Young, J., Swanson, G., West, D., et al. (1996). *Racial/ethnic patterns of cancer in the United States, 1988–1992.* Washington, DC: National Institutes of Health.

Mills, M., & Sullivan, K. (1999). The importance of information giving for patients newly diagnosed with cancer: A review of the literature. *Journal of Clinical Nursing, 8,* 631–642.

Morris, A., Billingsley, K., Baxter, N., & Baldwin, L. (2004). Racial disparities in rectal cancer treatment: A population-based analysis. *Archives of Surgery, 139*(2), 151–155.

Morrison, V., Picozzi, V., Scott, S., Pohlman, B., Dickman, E., Lee, M., et al. (2001). The impact of age on delivered dose intensity and hospitalizations for febrile neutropenia in patients with intermediate grade NHL receiving initial CHOP chemotherapy: A risk factor analysis. *Clinical Lymphoma, 2,* 47–56.

Murthy, V.H., Krumholz, H.M., & Gross, C.P. (2004). Participation in cancer clinical trials: Race-, sex-, and age-based disparities. *JAMA, 291,* 2720–2726.

Muss, H. (2001). Factors used to select adjuvant therapy of breast cancer in the United States: An overview of age, race and socioeconomic status. *Journal of the National Cancer Institute, 30,* 52–55.

National Cancer Institute. (2005). *Cancer health disparities: Fact sheet.* Retrieved January 15, 2006, from http://www.cancer.gov/cancertopics/factsheet/cancerhealthdisparities

Neugut, A., Garbowski, G., Lee, W., Murray, T., Nieves, J.W., Forde, K.A., et al. (1993). Dietary risk factors for the incidence and recurrence of colorectal adenomatous polyps: A case control study. *Annals of Internal Medicine, 118,* 91–95.

Neugut, A., Jacobson, J., & DeVivo, I. (1993). Epidemiology of colorectal adenomatous polyps. *Cancer Epidemiology, Biomarkers and Prevention, 2,* 159–176.

Nielesen-Bohlman, L., Panzer, A., & Kindig, D. (2004). *Institute of Medicine report: Health literacy: A prescription to end confusion.* Washington, DC: National Academies Press.

Norat, T., Lukanova, A., Ferrari, P., & Riboli, E. (2002). Meat consumption and colorectal cancer risk: Dose-response meta-analysis of epidemiological studies. *International Journal of Cancer, 98,* 241–256.

Peters, U., Sinha, R., Chatterjee, N., Subar, A.F., Ziegler, R.G., Kulldorff, M., et al. (2003). Dietary fibre and colorectal adenoma in a colorectal cancer early detection programme. *Lancet, 361,* 1491–1495.

Pisters, P., Kelsen, D., Powell, S., & Tepper, J. (2005). Cancer of the stomach. In V.T. DeVita, S. Hellman, & S. Rosenberg (Eds.), *Cancer: Principles and practice of oncology* (7th ed., pp. 909–944). Philadelphia: Lippincott Williams & Wilkins.

Platz, E.A., Willett, W.C., Colditz, G.A., Rimm, E.B., Spiegelman, D., & Giovannucci, E. (2000). Proportion of colon cancer risk that might be preventable in a cohort of middle-aged U.S. men. *Cancer Causes and Control, 11,* 579–588.

Posner, M., Forastiere, A., & Minsky, B. (2005). Cancer of the esophagus. In V.T. DeVita, S. Hellman, & S. Rosenberg (Eds.), *Cancer: Principles and practice of oncology* (7th ed., pp. 861–909). Philadelphia: Lippincott Williams & Wilkins.

Potosky, A., Harlan, L., Kaplan, R., Johnson, K., & Lynch, C. (2002). Age, sex and racial differences in the use of standard adjuvant therapy for colorectal cancer. *Journal of Clinical Oncology, 20,* 1192–1202.

Proctor, B., & Dalaker, J. (2003). *Poverty in the United States: 2002.* Washington, DC: U.S. Government Printing Office.

Rosen, A., & Schneider, E. (2004). Colorectal cancer screening disparities related to obesity and gender. *Journal of General Internal Medicine, 19,* 332–338.

Ryan, D., Compton, C., & Mayer, R. (2000). Carcinoma of the anal canal. *New England Journal of Medicine, 342,* 792–800.

Sandler, R.S., Halabi, S., Baron, J.A., Budinger, S., Paskett, E., Keresztes, R., et al. (2003). A randomized trial of aspirin to prevent colorectal adenomas in patients with previous colorectal cancer. *New England Journal of Medicine, 348,* 883–890.

Sargent, D.J., Goldberg, R.M., Jacobson, S.D., Macdonald, J.S., Labianca, R., Haller, D.G., et al. (2001). A pooled analysis of adjuvant chemotherapy for resected colon cancer in elderly patients. *New England Journal of Medicine, 345,* 1091–1097.

Schatzkin, A., Lanza, E., Corle, D., Lance, P., Iber, F., Caan, B., et al. (2000). Lack of effect of a low-fat high-fiber diet on the recurrence of colorectal adenomas. Polyp prevention trial study group. *New England Journal of Medicine, 342,* 1149–1155.

Shavers, V., & Brown, M.L. (2002). Racial and ethnic disparities in the receipt of cancer treatment. *Journal of the National Cancer Institute, 94,* 334–357.

Skalla, K., Bakitas, M., Furstenberg, D., Ahles, T., & Henderson, J. (2004). Patients' need for information about cancer therapy. *Oncology Nursing Forum, 31,* 313–319.

Smalley, W., Ray, W., Daugherty, J., & Griffin, M.R. (1999). Use of nonsteroidal anti-inflammatory drugs and incidence of colorectal cancer: A population-based study. *Archives of Internal Medicine, 159,* 161–166.

Smedley, B., Stite, A., & Nelson, A. (2002). *Unequal treatment: Confronting racial and ethnic disparities in health care.* Washington, DC: National Academies Press.

Steinbach, G., Lynch, P.M., Phillips, R.K.S., Wallace, M.H., Hawk, E., Gordon, G.B., et al. (2000). The effect of celecoxib, a cyclo-oxygenase-2 inhibitor, in familial adenomatous polyposis. *New England Journal of Medicine, 342,* 1946–1952.

Sturmer, T., Glynn, R., Lee, I.M., Manson, J.E., Buring, J.E., & Hennekens, C.H. (1998). Aspirin use and colorectal cancer: Post-trial follow-up data from the physicians' health study. *Annals of Internal Medicine, 128,* 713–720.

Talarico, L., Chen, G., & Pazdur, R. (2004). Enrollment of elderly patients in clinical trials for cancer drug registration: A 7-year experience by the U.S. Food and Drug Administration. *Journal of Clinical Oncology, 22,* 4626–4631.

Terry, M., Neugut, A., Bostick, R., Sandler, R.S., Haile, R.W., Jacobson, J.S., et al. (2002). Risk factors for advanced colorectal adenomas: A pooled analysis. *Cancer Epidemiology, Biomarkers and Prevention, 11,* 622–629.

Terry, P., Miller, A.B., & Rohan, T.E. (2002). Obesity and colorectal cancer risk in women. *Gut, 51*(2), 191–194.

Thun, M.J., Calle, E.E., Namboodiri, M.M., Flanders, W.D., Coates, R.J., Byers, T., et al. (1992). Risk factors for fatal colon cancer in a large prospective study. *Journal of the National Cancer Institute, 84,* 1491–1500.

Thun, M.J., Namboodiri, M.M., Calle, E.E., Flanders, W.D., & Heath, C.W., Jr. (1993). Aspirin use and risk of fatal cancer. *Cancer Research, 53,* 1322–1327.

Thun, M.J., Namboodiri, M.M., & Heath, C.W., Jr. (1991). Aspirin use and reduced risk of fatal colon cancer. *New England Journal of Medicine, 325,* 1593–1596.

Underwood, S., Powe, B., Canales, M., Meade, C., & Im, E. (2004). Cancer in U.S. ethnic and racial minority populations. *Annual Review of Nursing Research, 22,* 217–263.

Van Cutsem, E., & Costa, F. (2005). Progress in adjuvant treatment of colon cancer: Has it influenced clinical practice? *JAMA, 294,* 2758–2759.

Wactawski-Wende, J., Kotchen, J., Anderson, G., Assaf, A., Brunner, R., O'Sullivan, M., et al. (2006). Calcium plus vitamin D supplementation and the risk of colorectal cancer. *New England Journal of Medicine, 354,* 684–696.

Wallace, K., Baron, J.A., Cole, B.F., Sandler, R.S., Karagas, M.R., Beach, M.A., et al. (2004). Effect of calcium supplementation on the risk of large bowel polyps. *Journal of the National Cancer Institute, 96,* 921–925.

Ward, E., Jemal, A., Cokkinides, V.E., Singh, G., Cardinex, C., Ghafoor, A., et al. (2004). Cancer disparities by race/ethnicity and socioeconomic status. *CA: A Cancer Journal for Clinicians, 54,* 78–93.

Wilkes, G. (2005). Colon, rectal, and anal cancers. In M.H. Frogge, C.H. Yarbro, & M. Goodman (Eds.), *Cancer nursing: Principles and practice* (6th ed., pp. 1155–1215). Sudbury, MA: Jones and Bartlett.

Willett, W.C. (2005). Diet and cancer: An evolving picture. *JAMA, 293,* 233–234.

Willett, W.C., Stampfer, M.J., Colditz, G.A., Rosner, B.A., & Speizer, F.E. (1990). Relation of meat, fat, and fiber intake to the risk of colon cancer in a prospective study among women. *New England Journal of Medicine, 323,* 1664–1672.

Williams, M., Baker, D., Parker, R., & Nurss, J. (1998). Relationship of functional health literacy to patients' knowledge of their chronic disease. *Archives of Internal Medicine, 158,* 166–172.

Williams, M., Parker, R., Baker, D., Parikh, N.S., Pitkin, K., Coates, W.C., et al. (1995). Inadequate functional health literacy among patients at two public hospitals. *JAMA, 274,* 1677–1682.

Winawer, S.J., Zauber, A.G., Gerdes, H., O'Brien, M.J., Gottlieb, L.S., Sternberg, S.S., et al. (1996). Risk of colorectal cancer in the families of patients with adenomatous polyps. *New England Journal of Medicine, 334,* 82–87.

Winawer, S.J., Zauber, A.G., Ho, M., O'Brien, M.J., Gottlieb, L.S., Sternberg, S.S., et al. (1993). Prevention of colorectal cancer by colonoscopic polypectomy. The National Polyp Study Workgroup. *New England Journal of Medicine, 329,* 1977–1981.

Wrigley, H., Roderick, P., George, S., Smith, J., Mullee, M., & Goddard, J. (2003). Inequalities in survival from colorectal cancer: A comparison of the impact of deprivation, treatment, and host factors on observed and cause specific survival. *Journal of Epidemiology and Community Health, 57,* 301–309.

Xiong, H.Q., & Ajani, J.A. (2004). Treatment of colorectal cancer metastasis: The role of chemotherapy. *Cancer Metastasis Reviews, 23*(1–2), 145–163.

CHAPTER 2

Anatomy and Physiology of the Gastrointestinal Tract

Joyce P. Griffin-Sobel, RN, PhD, AOCN®, APRN,BC

Introduction

The gastrointestinal (GI) tract is a passageway from the mouth, through the esophagus, stomach, small and large intestines, and rectum leading to the anus (see Figure 2-1). It exists to ingest, digest, and eliminate food. The walls of the GI tract are, from the inside out, the mucosa, submucosa, muscularis, and serosa. Nerve stimuli come through local fibers, the enteric nervous system, and the autonomic nervous system by way of the enteric plexus. Muscular and autonomic activity of the GI tract helps to regulate motility, secretions, and blood flow.

Esophagus

The mouth is the entry for the GI tract, where food is mechanically chewed and mixed with saliva. Saliva is a watery substance mixed with mucus, electrolytes, and enzymes, such as alpha-amylase, which helps to initiate the digestion of carbohydrates (Huether, 2006). The esophagus is a hollow tube of approximately 10 inches (~25 cm) from the cricopharyngeus to the stomach and is composed of muscular layers (see Figure 2-2). It is flat unless distended by food. The esophagus has a sphincter at its proximal end, the cricopharyngeal muscle, which prevents air from gaining access to the esophagus during inspiration. The distal end of the esophagus contains the cardiac, or inferior, sphincter, which prevents food from moving backward from the stomach. Innervation of the esophagus is by motor neurons in the upper esophagus, with vagal stimulation in the lower aspect.

The esophagus bridges the neck, thorax, and abdomen as it moves food from the mouth to the stomach by peristalsis, which consists of a series of contractions of the muscular layers of the esophagus. The changes in wall tension occur from food stretching the muscular layers of the esophagus and stimulate peristalsis.

Figure 2-1. Anatomy of the Gastrointestinal System

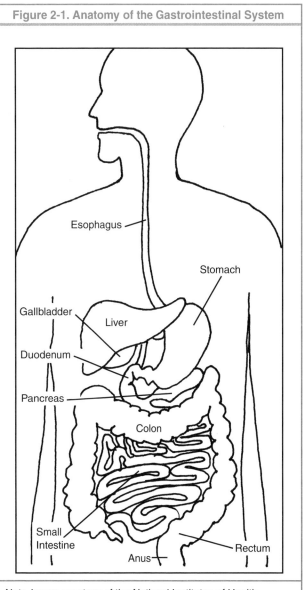

Note. Image courtesy of the National Institutes of Health.

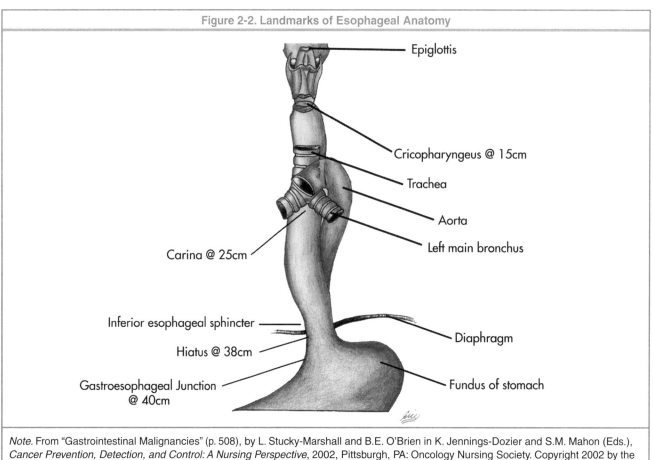

Figure 2-2. Landmarks of Esophageal Anatomy

- Epiglottis
- Cricopharyngeus @ 15cm
- Trachea
- Aorta
- Left main bronchus
- Carina @ 25cm
- Inferior esophageal sphincter
- Hiatus @ 38cm
- Gastroesophageal Junction @ 40cm
- Diaphragm
- Fundus of stomach

Note. From "Gastrointestinal Malignancies" (p. 508), by L. Stucky-Marshall and B.E. O'Brien in K. Jennings-Dozier and S.M. Mahon (Eds.), *Cancer Prevention, Detection, and Control: A Nursing Perspective*, 2002, Pittsburgh, PA: Oncology Nursing Society. Copyright 2002 by the Oncology Nursing Society. Reprinted with permission.

Swallowing

Most people think little about swallowing, unless a problem occurs. The act is a complex process, controlled by the swallowing center in the brain, the reticular formation in the brain stem, and the cerebellum. Cranial nerve functions, particularly the trigeminal (V), glossopharyngeal (IX), vagus (X), and hypoglossal (XII), also are essential to the swallowing process (Porth, 2005). The voluntary phase begins when the tongue forms a bolus of food, moving it back toward the pharynx. When the bolus of food enters the oropharynx, the involuntary, pharyngeal phase of swallowing begins. Respiration is coordinated with the swallowing movements to prevent food from entering the trachea, and the epiglottis moves posteriorly to cover and protect the larynx during the pharyngeal phase of swallowing.

During the esophageal phase of swallowing, the esophagus receives the food bolus in a series of peristaltic waves that move it downward. The cardiac sphincter, between the esophagus and stomach, relaxes prior to the onset of a contraction and returns to its resting state after food moves into the stomach. If the bolus of food does not pass at the usual pace through the esophagus, a second series of peristaltic waves will ensue, stimulated by the muscular wall distention (Huether, 2006; Lockhart & Resick,

2006). The inferior esophageal sphincter is controlled by the vagus nerve, and parasympathetic stimulation and the hormone gastrin increase the contraction of the sphincter.

Stomach

The stomach is a muscular, hollow organ that stores food, produces a number of digestive secretions, and partially digests food. Cells in the gastric mucosa produce digestive secretions, hormones, mucus, and enzymes. Parietal cells in the gastric glands secrete hydrochloric acid and intrinsic factor. Other gastric cells, the chief cells, secrete pepsinogen, which converts to the enzyme pepsin. G cells secrete gastrin, which is stimulated by protein in the stomach and prompts the secretion of hydrochloric acid (Huether, 2006). It lies in the upper abdomen, just under the diaphragm and the left lobe of the liver and above the transverse colon. It can accommodate almost 1,000 ml of contents. Food enters the stomach from the lower esophageal sphincter through the gastroduodenal junction, or the cardiac orifice. The distal orifice is the pyloric sphincter, which relaxes as food passes into the duodenum. The stomach has three areas: the fundus, or the upper portion, the body, and the antrum, or

Figure 2-3. Anatomic Landmarks of the Stomach

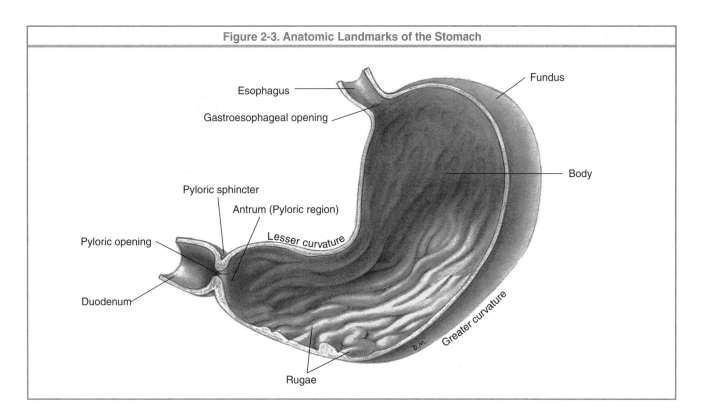

lower section (see Figure 2-3). The muscularis layer of the stomach has three layers of smooth muscle, which are thicker in the body and antrum to aid in the mixing of food as it moves into the duodenum. The blood supply from the celiac artery is abundant, as is the lymphatic drainage. Innervation is via the sympathetic and parasympathetic arms of the autonomic nervous system (Huether; Porth, 2005). Sympathetic stimuli enter the stomach through the celiac plexus, and parasympathetic stimuli enter through the vagus nerve. The enteric nervous system, which is within the GI tract, is active in controlling GI function. Two plexuses, the myenteric (Auerbach) and submucosal (Meissner), extend along the length of the GI tract. The neurons within these plexuses are regulated by a number of factors, such as local and hormonal stimuli or input from the autonomic nervous system, and they serve to control intestinal motility, coordination of intestinal segments, secretions, and absorption. Very little absorption occurs in the stomach, other than water, alcohol, and aspirin (Porth).

Stomach Functions

The stomach is active in mixing food with digestive juices, which it accomplishes by a process called retropulsion. Food moves toward the pyloric sphincter via peristalsis, but then is repetitively pushed backward toward the body of the stomach to mechanically break down food. Partially digested food, or chyme, passes into the duodenum in small amounts with each of these mechanical waves. The rate with which the stomach empties is dependent on volume, osmotic pressure,

and the characteristics of the stomach contents. The stomach secretes large volumes of gastric juices when eating begins, approximately 2,000 ml daily. Substances such as enzymes, hormones, intrinsic factor, gastroferrin, mucus, and acid are secreted. Gastric acid serves to dissolve food and destroy ingested microorganisms and is stimulated by the vagus nerve, gastrin, and histamine. Gastrin stimulates gastric acid secretion and leads to histamine release, which contributes to acid production. Acid is produced in the parietal cells, one of the gastric glands. Parietal cells also produce intrinsic factor, which allows for absorption of vitamin B_{12}. Gastroferrin aids in the absorption of iron. Pepsinogen, which becomes pepsin, is secreted and aids in protein digestion (Heuther, 2006; Porth, 2005).

Large quantities of food increase the rate of peristalsis and rate of emptying, whereby fats and nonisotonic matter delays emptying, by hormonal and neural mechanisms. The hormones gastrin and motilin, which are produced in the small intestine, stimulate gastric emptying. The stomach secretes cholecystokinin, which stimulates pancreatic enzymes and gastric inhibitory peptide, both inhibitors of gastric emptying, when chyme and fats are in the duodenum. This prevents fat from accumulating in the duodenum before bile is produced to digest it. Cholecystokinin stimulates the gallbladder to contract and discharge its bile into the duodenum. Similarly, osmoreceptors are activated in the duodenum to slow food passage (Huether, 2006; Porth, 2005).

Numerous conditions can affect gastric motility. Obstruction, hypertrophic pyloric stenosis, neuropathy, unpleasant odors and tastes, and fear all can slow gastric motility and inhibit gastric secretion. Similarly, aggression and hostility may trigger increased secretions and motility, and surgical procedures may disrupt vagal activity. Abnormally fast gastric emptying causes dumping syndrome (Porth, 2005; Smith & Morton, 2001).

Small Intestine

The small intestine is approximately 24 feet (~731 cm) in length and is composed of the duodenum, jejunum, and ileum (see Figure 2-4). The duodenum begins at the pylorus and joins the jejunum at the ligament of Treitz. Bile and pancreatic enzymes enter the GI tract in the duodenum. The jejunum and ileum are responsible for most nutrient absorption. The ileum terminates in the ileocecal valve, which controls flow into the colon from the ileum. The peritoneum, consisting of the visceral and parietal components, is a serous membrane around the organs of the abdomen. Visceral peritoneum covers the organs, whereas the parietal peritoneum lines the abdominal wall. The duodenum lies

behind the peritoneum, and the jejunum and ileum lie in the mesentery, a membrane fold attaching various organs to the body cavity or the peritoneum, which contains blood and lymphatic vessels supplying the intestine. The greater omentum, another fold of the peritoneum, covers most of the colon and can stop the spread of infection by adhering to the area of inflammation. The small intestine's blood supply is from the gastroduodenal and superior mesenteric arteries, and similar to the rest of the GI tract, it is innervated by sympathetic and parasympathetic fibers. The sympathetic fibers inhibit motility, whereas parasympathetic stimuli control secretion, motility, and pain sensation.

Nutrient absorption is accomplished through villi, finger-like projections of mucous membrane that line the entire small intestine and secrete necessary enzymes (see Figure 2-5). They are composed of enterocytes and goblet cells, which secrete mucus, and these cells adhere to each other at junctions where water and electrolytes are absorbed. Each villus has an artery, vein, and lymph vessel that allow maximal blood flow for transport and absorption of nutrients. Microvilli are tiny projections that create the brush border, increasing the absorptive area and secreting digestive enzymes. Crypts of Lieberkuhn

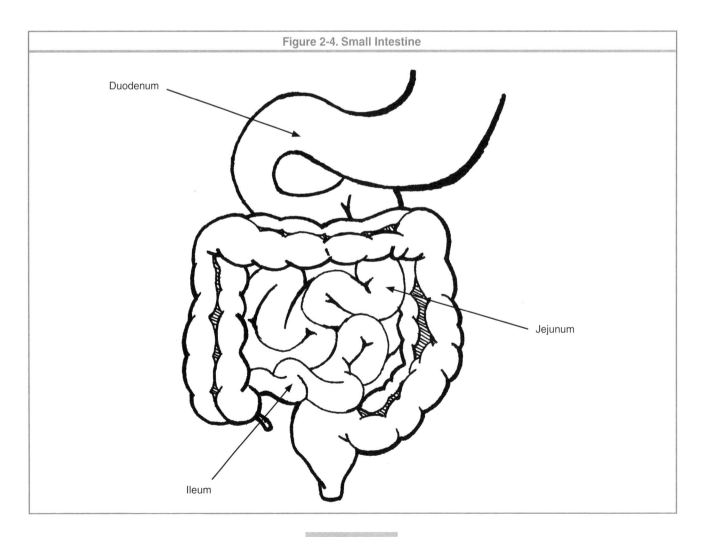

Figure 2-4. Small Intestine

Duodenum

Jejunum

Ileum

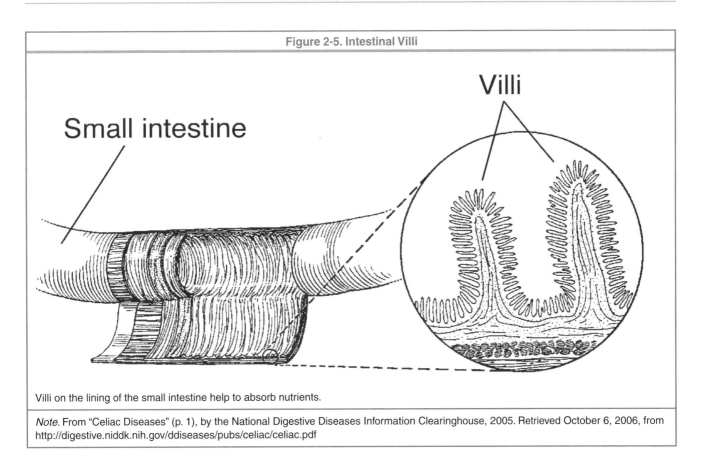

Figure 2-5. Intestinal Villi

Villi on the lining of the small intestine help to absorb nutrients.

Note. From "Celiac Diseases" (p. 1), by the National Digestive Diseases Information Clearinghouse, 2005. Retrieved October 6, 2006, from http://digestive.niddk.nih.gov/ddiseases/pubs/celiac/celiac.pdf

are located between the bases of villi and produce the stem cells of the enterocytes that arise from the base of the crypt and move out to the tip of the villus as they mature. Starvation, vitamin B_{12} deficiency, cytotoxic drugs, and irradiation all can shorten villi (Huether, 2006; Porth, 2005).

The duodenum is primarily responsible for absorption of iron, calcium, fats, sugars, proteins, vitamins, and water. The jejunum absorbs sugars and protein, and the ileum absorbs bile salts, vitamin B_{12}, and chloride. Water-soluble vitamins, such as the B vitamins and C, are absorbed in the small intestine. Fat-soluble vitamins, A, D, E, and K, also are absorbed there (Huether, 2006). Pancreatic fluid drains into the duodenum. The pancreas consists of clusters of endocrine cells, the islets of Langerhans, and other cells that produce enzymes and hormones, such as amylase, trypsin, and lipase, all of which contribute to protein, fat, and carbohydrate digestion and absorption. Cholecystokinin controls pancreatic secretion that stimulates the release of digestive enzymes and secretin, which affects the release of bicarbonate (Porth, 2005; Smith & Morton, 2001).

Large Intestine

The large intestine is four to five feet (122–152 cm) long, with a diameter of about two to three inches. It consists of the cecum, appendix, colon, rectum, and anal canal (see Figure 2-6). Chyme, material produced by gastric digestion of food, is passed from the ileum to the cecum, a blind pouch that has the appendix attached to it. The appendix has no known function. The colon, divided into the ascending, transverse, descending, and sigmoid colon, ends in the rectum. The ileocecal valve is the sphincter that controls the inflow of chyme from the ileum to the cecum, and the O'Beirne sphincter controls flow from the sigmoid colon into the rectum. The rectum is divided into three sections: the lower rectum, which is 3–6 cm from the anal verge (the distal end of the anal canal); the upper rectum, which is 10–15 cm above the anal verge; and the midrectum, which is in between. The mesorectum is a fold of peritoneum or mesentery attached to the rectum. The anal canal is the terminal part of the large intestine, situated between the anal verge and the rectum. It is approximately 2–4 cm long and extends to the anus, the external opening. A thick layer of smooth muscle surrounds the anal canal, forming the internal sphincter, and overlapping muscle forms the external anal sphincter. The internal anal sphincter contracts until it reflexively relaxes when the rectum is distended (see Figure 2-7). Innervation of the large intestine is similar to the small intestine: sympathetic stimuli modulate intestinal reflexes, relay sensations of pain or fullness, and control the defecation reflex. Parasympathetic stimuli affect motility. Blood

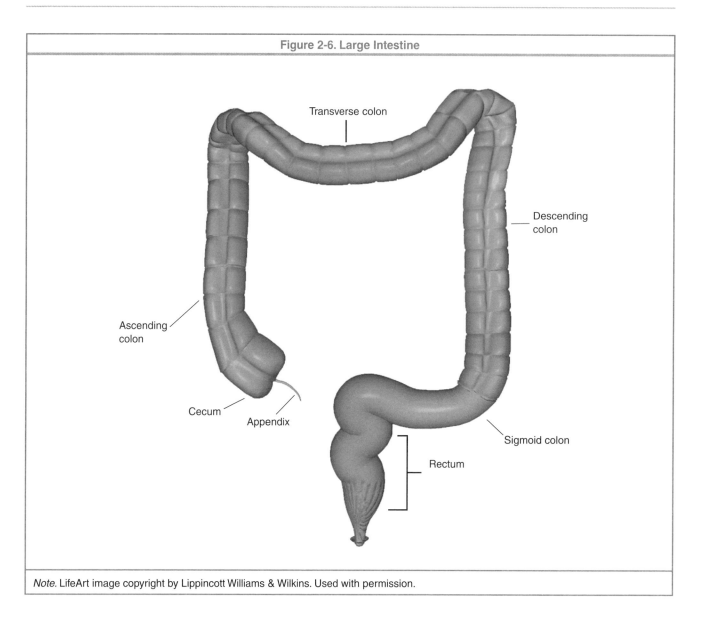

Figure 2-6. Large Intestine

Transverse colon

Descending colon

Ascending colon

Cecum

Appendix

Sigmoid colon

Rectum

Note. LifeArt image copyright by Lippincott Williams & Wilkins. Used with permission.

supply of the large intestine and rectum is from the superior and inferior mesenteric artery.

The mucosa of the colon contains columnar epithelial cells, which absorb fluid and electrolytes, goblet cells, which produce mucus, and crypts of Lieberkuhn. Abnormal crypts of the colon have been identified as possible precursors of adenomas and cancer, especially those crypts that are larger and have dysplastic features (Takayama et al., 1998). The colon contains an enormous population of microorganisms, primarily anaerobes such as *Bacteroides,* clostridia, and coliforms. At birth, the intestinal tract is sterile, but after three to four weeks, normal flora is present. These microorganisms play a role in bile salt metabolism. There are no villi in the large intestine (Huether, 2006; Porth, 2005).

The colon receives liquid residue after the small intestine digests and absorbs all possible nutrients. Primarily water and nondigestible material, such as cellulose, are passed to the colon. Reabsorption of water is the chief function of the colon by active transport and diffusion. By the time the residue reaches the sigmoid, the waste matter is solid feces. Movement occurs when the circular muscles contract at different sites within the colon, moving the contents back and forth. The defecation reflex, or rectal reflex, is stimulated by stretching within the rectum and can be voluntarily suppressed. When the internal anal sphincter relaxes, and if the person voluntarily relaxes the external sphincter, defecation occurs.

Summary

The ingestion and digestion of nutrients requires a sophisticated coordination system. Disorders of function such as Hirschsprung disease, which leads to megacolon from

Figure 2-7. Anatomy of the Anus

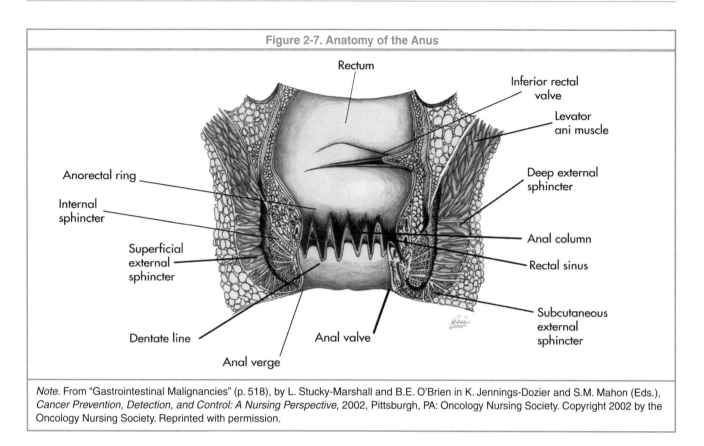

Note. From "Gastrointestinal Malignancies" (p. 518), by L. Stucky-Marshall and B.E. O'Brien in K. Jennings-Dozier and S.M. Mahon (Eds.), *Cancer Prevention, Detection, and Control: A Nursing Perspective,* 2002, Pittsburgh, PA: Oncology Nursing Society. Copyright 2002 by the Oncology Nursing Society. Reprinted with permission.

constipation, or dumping syndrome, where intestinal contents move too rapidly, demonstrate the importance of synchronized movement within the colon. Any dysfunction within the GI tract can lead to nutritional deficiencies, inflammatory processes, disorders of elimination, and significant patient distress. Having a comprehensive knowledge of GI anatomy and physiology will aid nurses in planning care for patients.

References

Huether, S. (2006). Structure and function of the digestive system. In K. McCance & S. Huether (Eds.), *Pathophysiology: The biologic basis for disease in adults and children* (5th ed., pp. 1353–1383). St. Louis, MO: Elsevier Mosby.

Lockhart, J., & Resick, L. (2006). Anatomy and physiology. In L. Clarke & M. Dropkin (Eds.), *Site-specific cancer series: Head and neck cancer* (pp. 5–16). Pittsburgh, PA: Oncology Nursing Society.

Porth, C. (2005). Control of gastrointestinal function. In C. Porth (Ed.), *Pathophysiology: Concepts of altered health states* (7th ed., pp. 871–884). Philadelphia: Lippincott Williams & Wilkins.

Smith, M., & Morton, D. (2001). *The digestive system.* St. Louis, MO: Elsevier Mosby.

Takayama, T., Katsuki, S., Takahashi, Y., Ohi, M., Nojiri, S., Sakamaki, S., et al. (1998). Aberrant crypt foci of the colon as precursors of adenoma and cancer. *New England Journal of Medicine, 339,* 1277–1284.

CHAPTER 3

Biology, Prevention, and Screening

Joyce P. Griffin-Sobel, RN, PhD, AOCN®, APRN,BC

Introduction

A significant number of deaths from gastrointestinal (GI) cancers are preventable with proper screening, for which a number of professional organizations have issued recommendations. Media coverage of Katie Couric's colonoscopy on national news had a large impact; however, the public continues to avoid screening. By educating patients that a polyp takes about a decade to grow and become malignant, healthcare professionals can help patients to understand that death from colorectal cancer (CRC), specifically, can be prevented. Oncology nurses have a professional obligation to promote screening to patients and the public. The Oncology Nursing Society has issued a position statement on prevention and early detection in the United States that highlights the importance of public and professional education and program evaluation (see Appendix A).

Biology

Colorectal Cancers

CRCs usually are adenocarcinomas and can be hereditary or sporadic in origin. Approximately 75% of people diagnosed with CRC have no risk factors. Individuals with a family history of CRC or adenomas are at greater risk of developing CRC. A first-degree relative with either CRC or adenoma increases the patient's risk by two- to threefold (National Cancer Institute [NCI], 2005). Approximately 20%–30% of CRCs may arise from an inherited predisposition, separate from the known hereditary cancers (Libutti, Saltz, Rustgi, & Tepper, 2005). For any individual who has been diagnosed earlier than age 45 or has two or more relatives with CRC, a genetic basis should be evaluated. In addition, a history of inflammatory bowel disease increases the personal risk of CRC (American Cancer Society [ACS], 2005b). Inherited colon cancers, which are approximately 6% of cases, are of two types: familial adenomatous polyposis (FAP) or hereditary nonpolyposis colorectal cancer (HNPCC).

Esophageal and Gastric Cancers

Esophageal cancers can be squamous cell carcinoma or adenocarcinoma, the latter showing an increased incidence in the United States. Barrett's esophagus, a progressive metaplasia of the distal esophagus, is a significant risk factor for developing adenocarcinoma of the esophagus and is caused by chronic gastric reflux (Stucky-Marshall & O'Brien, 2002). Numerous reports over the past 50 years have linked gastroesophageal reflux disease (GERD) to Barrett's esophagus or esophageal adenocarcinoma (Reid, 2005). However, it is important to note that the vast majority of patients with GERD or Barrett's esophagus do not progress to cancer during their lifetimes (Reid). The majority of adenocarcinomas are in the distal esophagus, and squamous cell carcinomas are distributed more often in the middle and distal esophageal sections (Enzinger & Mayer, 2003) (see Figure 3-1). Gastric cancers usually are adenocarcinoma and, less commonly, squamous cell carcinoma (Stucky-Marshall & O'Brien).

Path to Carcinogenesis

Most CRCs arise from adenomatous polyps in the colon, and the process of carcinogenesis has been extensively studied. Polyps can be neoplastic, such as the adenomatous polyps, which can become malignant; hyperplastic, which do not have malignant potential; or submucosal lesions (Macrae & Young, 1999). Adenomatous polyps, or adenomas, have three types: pedunculated—stalked or tubular, sessile—flat or villous, and combination—tubulovillous.

Tubular adenomas, approximately 80% of adenomas, are attached to the mucosal surface by a stalk. Sessile adenomas constitute 3%–16% of adenomas and typically are found in the rectosigmoid colon. They usually are broad-based, elevated lesions with a cauliflower-like surface. Tubulovillous adenomas (8%–16% of polyps) are a cross between the two (Porth, 2005). The majority of adenomas are polypoid, but 20%–30% of them are flat or depressed (Walsh & Terdiman, 2003). The prevalence

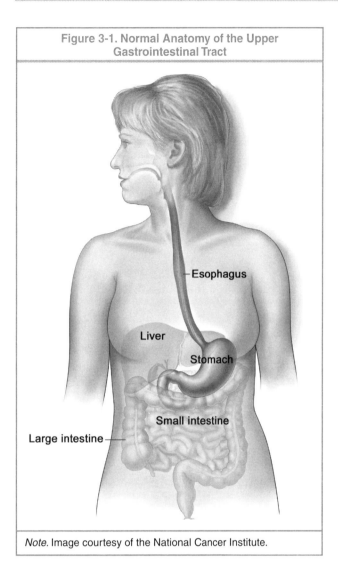

Figure 3-1. Normal Anatomy of the Upper Gastrointestinal Tract

Esophagus

Liver

Stomach

Small intestine

Large intestine

Note. Image courtesy of the National Cancer Institute.

The increasing incidence of obesity is thought to be a significant factor in the development of esophageal cancer because of its relationship to GERD (Enzinger & Mayer). Gastric cancers also are thought to be secondary to irritation or infection, especially *Helicobacter pylori*, which increases the risk three- to sixfold. Polyps are uncommon in the stomach, but when they occur, they should be removed, as 11% will develop malignant changes (Stucky-Marshall & O'Brien, 2002).

Genetics in Colorectal Carcinomas

A series of genetic and cellular functions regulate carcinogenesis and have been described extensively. Proto-oncogenes, normal cellular genes, become oncogenes when inappropriately or excessively activated (Merkle & Loescher, 2005) (see Figure 3-2). An oncogene is capable of turning a normal cell into a malignant one. Growth factors are a type of oncogene that interact with a specific receptor to alter expression of certain genes, or signaling. Several growth factors, when overproduced, are linked to cancer. Vascular endothelial growth factor, the most well-known growth factor of angiogenesis, is important in the development of a blood supply to a tumor.

High microvascular density correlates with angiogenic activity and is associated with poor prognosis after resection (Poon, Fun, & Wong, 2003). Microvessel density is proportional to the vascular endothelial growth factor content of the tumor. Growth factor receptors, most of which possess tyrosine kinase activity, release signals into the cell, which stimulates mitotic division and cell proliferation. Various growth factor receptors have been implicated in the pathology of CRC (Loescher & Whitesell, 2003). Epidermal growth factor receptor (EGFR) is one type of an oncogene where overexpression inhibits apoptosis (Merkle & Loescher, 2005) and correlates with poor prognosis in several malignancies. CRC cells overexpress EGFR. The U.S. Food and Drug Administration has approved cetuximab, an antibody directed against EGFR, for treatment of CRC (Dannenberg, Lippman, Mann, Subbaramaiah, & DuBois, 2005). However, if a tumor is negative for EGFR by immunohistochemistry, it does not rule out a response to cetuximab (Chung et al., 2005).

Signal transducers are proteins that activate the growth factor receptors in the cell. One example is the *Ras* superfamily, which acts to regulate cell proliferation and differentiation. Activation of *Ras* by mutation is frequent in cancers of the colon, lung, and pancreas, and *K-ras* mutations commonly are found in tumors of the colon. Tumor suppressor genes, the genes controlling proto-oncogene activity, are abnormal in many CRCs. The genes identified to date include the *APC*, *DCC* (deleted in colon cancer), *MLH1*, *MLH2*, and *TP53*. Mutations of *TP53*, in particular, are common in many cancers. Apoptosis, or programmed cell death, may be negatively affected by *TP53* mutation, resulting in rapid tumor progression (Loescher & Whitesell, 2003). EGFR overexpression, caused

of adenomatous polyps increases with age, rising to 40%–50% by age 60, and affects men and women equally (Porth). Colorectal adenomas are premalignant lesions that increase one's risk for developing CRC. Aberrant crypt foci, or crypt-like lesions in the colonic wall, are being evaluated as possible precursors to adenoma formation (Takayama et al., 1998). The path from normal colonic mucosa to adenomatous polyp to CRC takes about 10 years and is strongly linked with several genetic alterations.

The etiology of esophageal cancer is unclear. Tobacco smoke, alcohol, or GERD may irritate and damage the esophagus and predispose an individual to squamous cell carcinoma, as does lower socioeconomic status (Enzinger & Mayer, 2003). GERD is linked to the development of adenocarcinoma of the esophagus, as are hiatal hernia, frequent use of antacids, and drinking extremely hot beverages (Enzinger & Mayer). Drugs that relax the sphincter at the gastroesophageal junction, such as beta-blockers, can increase the risk for adenocarcinoma of the esophagus. A history of radiotherapy to the chest also predisposes the patient to esophageal cancer (Enzinger & Mayer).

Figure 3-2. Colon Carcinogenesis and the Effects of Chemopreventive Agents

Proposed sequence of molecular genetic events in the evolution of colon cancer. Carcinomas arise from an accumulation of events whose sequence has been defined. Alterations in *APC* or DNA mismatch repair genes may be inherited in the germline (familial adenomatous polyposis, HNPCC) or may be acquired after birth (somatic mutations). Bottom row (A–C), histology. Top row (D–F), colonoscopic photographs. From left to right: Dysplastic aberrant crypt focus (A, D with methylene blue staining), adenomatous polyp (B, E), and invasive carcinoma (C, F). [From Takayama et al. (1998). Aberrant crypt foci of the colon as precursors of adenoma and cancer. *New England Journal of Medicine, 339,* 1277.]

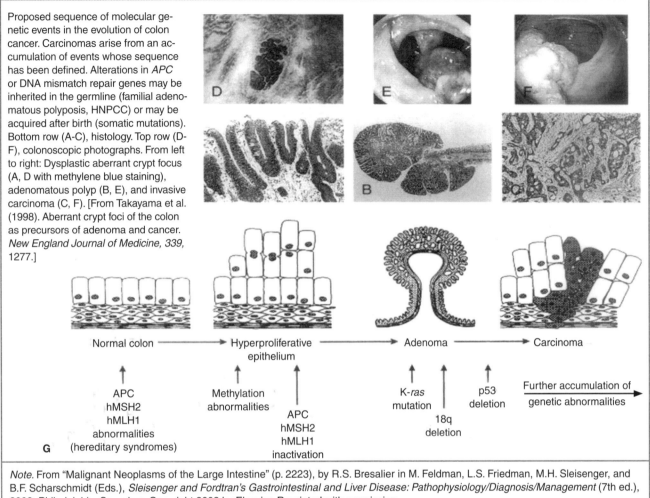

Note. From "Malignant Neoplasms of the Large Intestine" (p. 2223), by R.S. Bresalier in M. Feldman, L.S. Friedman, M.H. Sleisenger, and B.F. Scharschmidt (Eds.), *Sleisenger and Fordtran's Gastrointestinal and Liver Disease: Pathophysiology/Diagnosis/Management* (7th ed.), 2002, Philadelphia: Saunders. Copyright 2002 by Elsevier. Reprinted with permission.

by inhibiting apoptosis, promotes angiogenesis and metastatic spread (Wilkes, 2005). The majority of CRCs arise from mutations in the *TP53*, *SMAD4*, and *APC* genes, which are tumor suppressor genes. Many polyps acquire additional mutations in the *Ras* oncogenes as they grow (Libutti et al., 2005).

A smaller percentage of CRCs arise through the microsatellite instability (MSI) pathway. Microsatellites are gene regions in which DNA sequences are repeated, and during replication, mutations can occur. The mutations result in contractions or lengthening, causing instability. Mismatch-repair proteins usually repair these mutations, but repair is difficult in tumors with a deficiency of the proteins. MSI is a marker of mismatch-repair deficiency and is found more frequently in cancers proximal to the splenic flexure, in both sporadic and inherited cancers, in those that are more often poorly differentiated, and those of a larger size. HNPCC tumors usually are characterized by a high-frequency MSI (MSI-H) phenotype, and patients frequently have a larger primary tumor

at diagnosis, have right-sided high-grade tumors, and have a good prognosis. Patients with CRC that exhibit MSI have a longer survival than those patients without it and respond differently to chemotherapy (Ribic et al., 2003). Fluorouracil-based chemotherapy appeared to be beneficial to patients with stage II or III colon cancer with microsatellite stable (MSS) tumors but not those with tumors exhibiting MSI-H (Ribic et al.). Chemotherapy in individuals with MSI-H does not significantly increase, and potentially may decrease, overall and disease-free survival. Sporadic CRC exhibits MSI infrequently (approximately 15% of cases), whereas those with HNPCC demonstrate MSI in approximately 87% of cases (Agrawal et al., 2005).

One rare familial genetic syndrome, tylosis, or an abnormality at chromosome 17, predisposes a patient to esophageal cancer. It predisposes the patient to a 95% risk of developing squamous cell cancer by 70 years of age (Enzinger & Mayer, 2003). Chromosomal losses are present in Barrett's esophageal adenocarcinomas that are poorly understood (Enzinger & Mayer).

Tumor markers are antigens expressed on the surface of a tumor, cells or substances released from normal cells in response to the presence of a tumor. They are used in screening, prognosticating, and monitoring treatment. Carcinoembryonic antigen (CEA) is the tumor marker used most frequently in CRC. GI mucosa normally expresses a small amount of this protein, and a normal CEA level is 2.5 ng/ml or less for nonsmokers and 5 ng/ml for smokers (Sweed & Meropol, 2001).

Hereditary Colorectal Cancers

The two major hereditary CRCs are FAP and Lynch syndrome, or HNPCC. FAP accounts for 1% of cases of CRC in the United States, and HNPCC for 5% (Winawer et al., 1996).

Hereditary Nonpolyposis Colorectal Cancer

A germ-line mutation in any of the mismatch-repair genes leads to HNPCC. This autosomal dominant CRC is the most common form of hereditary colon cancer and comprises 5% of all CRCs (Douglas et al., 2005). The pedigree reveals instances of early onset CRC (mean age 45 years) and more right-sided tumors, which usually are proximal to the splenic flexure (Lynch & de la Chapelle, 2003). HNPCC has a number of characteristic features (Lynch & de la Chapelle):

- Early age at diagnosis of CRC, usually by age 45
- Pattern of primary cancers within the pedigree, such as colonic and endometrial cancer
- Survival different from the norm, with a better long-term prognosis than patients with MSS tumors
- Poorly differentiated tumors with accelerated progression to cancer
- Identification of a germ-line mutation in affected members.

HNPCC cancers are more likely to be right-sided and mucinous, possess MSI, and behave less aggressively. Patients present with a larger tumor than with MSS tumors, which are the majority of CRCs. In HNPCC I (or Lynch syndrome I), tumors may develop from multiple and flat polyps, with more rapid progression from adenoma to carcinoma. Mean age for CRC is 45 years. MSI from mutations in mismatch-repair genes, or MSI-H, is found in almost all HNPCC cancers (Lynch & de la Chapelle, 2003).

In HNPCC II (Lynch syndrome II), other cancers, particularly endometrial, ovarian, stomach (especially in Korea and Japan), small bowel, pancreas, brain, hepatobiliary, and uroepithelial tract, are seen (Lynch & de la Chapelle, 2003). Risk for development of CRC in HNPCC is 70%–90%, endometrial cancer is 40%–60%, and ovarian cancer is 10%–12% (Libutti et al., 2005). One study found prophylactic hysterectomies and bilateral salpingo-oopho-

rectomies were effective in preventing endometrial and ovarian cancers in women with Lynch syndrome (Schmeler et al., 2006).

Diagnoses of HNPCC syndromes are based on two sets of criteria, the Amsterdam II criteria and the revised Bethesda guidelines. The Amsterdam II criteria are

- At least three relatives with HNPCC-associated cancers (colorectal, endometrial, small bowel, ureter, or renal pelvis)
- At least two successive generations are affected.
- At least one case before age 50
- FAP is excluded.
- Histopathologic verification of tumors (Libutti et al., 2005).

Amsterdam I criteria defined the syndrome of HNPCC as above, with the exception of associated cancers. Amsterdam II expanded the criteria to include extracolonic cancers (Garber & Offit, 2005).

The Bethesda criteria include molecular genetic considerations and are used to identify patients whose colorectal tumors should be tested for MIS (Umar et al., 2004).

- CRC diagnosed before the age of 50
- Presence of synchronous, metachronous, colorectal, or other HNPCC-associated tumors (CRC, endometrial, stomach, ovarian, pancreas, ureter, renal pelvis, biliary tract)
- CRC with MSI-H histology diagnosed in a patient younger than 60
- CRC diagnosed in one or more first-degree relative(s) with an HNPCC-related tumor, with one of the cancers being diagnosed before age 50
- CRC diagnosed in two or more first- or second-degree relatives with HNPCC-related tumors, regardless of age

Annual colonoscopies are recommended in these patients, because adenomas progress rapidly to cancer. Screening should begin at 20–25 years of age (Garber & Offit, 2005). Screening for other cancers, especially endometrial and ovarian, also is recommended.

Familial Adenomatous Polyposis

FAP is a hereditary disorder caused by the inheritance of a mutated copy of the adenomatosis polyposis coli *(APC)* gene, which leads to polyposis at an early age (Libutti et al., 2005). To date, only one FAP gene has been discovered, but more than 300 different mutations have been identified (National Human Genome Research Institute, 2005). These individuals have an accelerated progression to CRCs, which are more likely to be distal; have *APC, p53,* and *K-ras* gene mutations; and be aggressive. Multiple adenomatous polyps that proliferate throughout the colon and develop at an early age characterize the disease. Risk for colon cancer is nearly 100%, and malignancy usually develops by age 40–50 (Lynch & de la Chapelle, 2003). Patients with an *APC* mutation or family members with FAP should be screened annually with a flexible sigmoidoscopy, starting at age 10–12. As the disease progresses, patients may require prophylactic subtotal colectomy. Cancers of the stomach also may occur, particularly in Korean and Japanese patients (Lynch & de la Chapelle).

Other features of the disease include desmoid formation, osteomas, and cysts. A desmoid tumor is a locally invasive, nonmetastasizing fibromatous tumor, which can grow aggressively. Genetic testing may be of value in identifying those patients likely to develop desmoids following surgery for any reason (NCI, 2005). The term *Gardner syndrome* refers to the soft tissue, bony, and dental abnormalities occurring in these families. Other tumors can occur, including pancreatic cancer, papillary thyroid carcinoma, sarcoma, and hepatoblastoma. *Turcot syndrome* refers to the occurrence of brain tumors, glioblastoma multiforme or medulloblastoma, with colonic polyposis (Libutti et al., 2005).

Duodenal adenomas are found in the majority of patients with FAP, resulting in a 4%–12% incidence of duodenal adenocarcinomas. The most definitive procedure for reducing the risk, without substantial morbidity, is pancreas-sparing duodenectomy (NCI, 2005).

People at high risk of FAP are screened annually for polyps, usually in early teenage years. Once a family member with FAP is diagnosed with polyposis, colectomy is recommended. Deciding the appropriate time for surgery depends on open and honest discussions with the patient and family members. Celecoxib at 400 mg twice a day, a cyclooxygenase (COX)-2 inhibitor, reduced the number of colorectal polyps compared to controls and was approved for polyp prevention in 2000 (Steinbach et al., 2000). Sulindac also reduces adenoma formation (Garber & Offit, 2005); however, polyps can return.

Patients who are suspected of having a familial, hereditary colon cancer should be referred to a genetic counselor for *APC* gene testing, which is commercially available. Women also need annual endometrial and ovarian cancer screening.

Screening

Screening decreases the incidence of CRC (Mandel et al., 2000). Annual fecal occult blood tests (FOBTs) reduce mortality from CRC by 33% and its incidence by 20% (Mandel et al., 1993; Mandel et al., 2000). If Americans adhered to screenings, more than 29,600 diagnoses of CRC could be avoided (Church et al., 2004). No recommended screening guidelines exist for esophageal, gastric, or anal cancers.

Colorectal Screening

ACS recommended that individuals 50 years of age and older who are at average risk begin screening for CRC by using one of the following techniques.

- Annual FOBT or fecal immunochemical test (FIT)
- Flexible sigmoidoscopy every five years
- Annual FOBT or FIT and flexible sigmoidoscopy every five years
- Colonoscopy every 10 years
- Double contrast barium enema (DCBE) every five years (ACS, 2005b).

More intense surveillance is recommended for individuals at increased risk who have

- A history of adenomatous polyps
- A history of curative resection of CRC
- A family history of CRC or colorectal adenomas diagnosed in a first-degree relative before age 60
- A history of inflammatory bowel disease of significant duration
- A family history or genetic testing indicating the presence of one of two hereditary syndromes (ACS, 2005b).

These guidelines are supported by the U.S. Multisociety Task Force on CRC, which recently updated its guidelines (Winawer et al., 2003), and numerous other professional organizations. Digital rectal exams are recommended annually, beginning at age 50, by the American Society of Colon and Rectal Surgeons (Mahon, 2004). However, one study found that digital rectal exams did not reduce mortality from rectal cancer (Herrinton, Selby, Friedman, Quesenberry, & Weiss, 1995). Medicare and most other health plans now provide coverage for CRC screening.

Fecal Occult Blood Test

FOBTs, which detect blood loss in the stool, should be performed annually beginning at age 50 (Mahon, 2004). The most commonly used test is the Hemoccult® II (Beckman-Coulter, Palo Alto, CA). The patient applies two samples of three different stools to test cards. When a developer substance of hydrogen peroxide is applied to the card, a blue color appears when positive. The more test windows that are positive, the greater the predictive value of the test (Walsh & Terdiman, 2003). Consumption of red meat, horseradish, and turnips can result in a false positive, and vitamin C can produce a false negative. A recent review questions these diet restrictions, concluding they may reduce patient compliance with screening but not reduce the positivity rate (Pignone, Campbell, Carr, & Phillips, 2001). Rehydration of the stool specimen results in higher false-positive rates and is not recommended by the U.S. Preventive Services Task Force and the World Health Organization (Walsh & Terdiman).

Flexible Sigmoidoscopy

Flexible sigmoidoscopy is performed with a 60-cm flexible endoscope after the patient receives a saline enema. A nurse can perform the procedure in an office setting with appropriate training. Sedation rarely is needed, and the patient may experience some abdominal cramping. Complication rates are extremely low. If a polyp larger than 1 cm or multiple polyps are found, the patient should have a full colonoscopy. Because only a small portion of the colon is examined during a sigmoidoscopy, adenomas or lesions in other parts of the colon will be missed. No randomized controlled trials have demonstrated the effectiveness of sigmoidoscopy in the prevention of CRC deaths (Walsh & Terdiman, 2003).

Colonoscopies were conducted at 13 Veterans Affairs (VA) Medical Centers on men who had three consecutive days of FOBTs. The study found that half of the advanced adenomas and colon cancer lesions were not detected after FOBTs and sigmoidoscopy as part of the colonoscopy (Lieberman et al., 2001).

Colonoscopy

An endoscopist or gastroenterologist, using a 160-cm flexible endoscope, performs a colonoscopy (see Figure 3-3). The patient preparation is significant: a clear liquid diet the day prior to the test and a purgative. The patient is sedated for the procedure, which takes about 30 minutes. Extensive training is required to perform the procedure safely and effectively (Marshall, 1995). The entire colon is visualized, extending to the cecum. Large cohort studies of individuals who had polyps removed during colonoscopy demonstrated a reduction in CRC incidence (Mandel et al., 1993; Winawer et al., 1993). The National Polyp Study showed a greater than 75% reduction in CRC after polyps were removed in a colonoscopy (Winawer et al., 2003). Colonoscopy is the most sensitive of the tests for detection of adenomas and cancers (Walsh & Terdiman, 2003). If a polyp is detected, the patient should have another colonoscopy in three to five years (Bond, 2000). If the colonoscopy is negative or no polyps are detected, the patient should repeat the procedure in 10 years. Colonoscopy is considered safe, with no deaths or colonic perforations directly attributable to the procedure in one large study (Lieberman et al., 2001). In studies of colonoscopy screening, complications of bleeding in one and stroke have been reported in 0.3% of subjects, and deaths have occured in three subjects within one month of colonoscopy (Walsh & Terdiman). However, infection rates after the procedure are unknown because no mandatory reporting mechanism exists.

Double Contrast Barium Enema

DCBE is a radiologic technique where barium and air are instilled into the colon after complete bowel preparation, similar to that of colonoscopy. The patient is moved into different positions on the examining table while radiographs are taken. No sedation is required, and the procedure has a very low complication rate. Although not as sensitive as a colonoscopy, DCBE detects a majority of advanced adenomas (Walsh & Terdiman, 2003). However, even for polyps 1 cm and larger, sensitivity is about 50%. One study compared colonoscopy with DCBE, and the latter did not detect many of the smaller lesions (Winawer et al., 2000). DCBE usually is performed in patients who are poor candidates for colonoscopy.

Emerging Screening Techniques

Virtual Colonoscopy

Virtual colonoscopy is a new technique that uses two- and three-dimensional views of the colon using computed tomography or magnetic resonance imaging. After a bowel preparation, as with colonoscopy, air is instilled into the colon and images are obtained. The procedure takes about five minutes. A radiologist then reviews the images. Patients must have a full colonoscopy if abnormalities are found with the virtual technique. Additionally, removal of polyps and biopsies cannot be performed with this technique. Nevertheless, patients often request it, assuming by the word "virtual" that little prep is needed. Good sensitivity for detection of large polyps has been reported, but questions remain about its reliability for lesions smaller than 1 cm (Walsh & Terdiman, 2003). Controversy exists about its accuracy because inter-rater variability has been reported (Johnson et al., 2003). Radiologists need extensive training in interpreting the images, and more data are needed about its accuracy and reliability before it can be recommended for widespread screening.

Stool-Based Screening

Immunochemical stool screening detects the intact globin protein segment of human hemoglobin. No dietary restrictions are needed prior to testing, and early studies estimate an 87% sensitivity for adenomas greater than 10 mm (Mahon, 2004). Fecal DNA stool tests also are being studied extensively. These tests detect as many as 19 genetic abnormalities, such as *K-ras* and *APC,* in fecal samples. Studies have reported 71%–92% of sensitivities (Dong et al., 2001).

Barriers to Screening

CRC screening is not something the public has embraced. Studies have estimated that screening rates by FOBT or endoscopic techniques within the past five years range from 39.5%–50% (ACS, 2005b; Mahon, 2004; Rosen & Schneider, 2004). Reasons include conflicts with work, access, embarrassment, fear, lack of a provider, and financial limitations.

African Americans report lower rates of screening with FOBT or colonoscopy than Caucasians, and the difference becomes greater with advancing age (Agrawal et al., 2005). Obese women also are less likely to undergo screening for CRC (Rosen & Schneider, 2004).

Studies have shown that education and reinforcement by providers will increase patient CRC screening. One study (Ferreira et al., 2005) targeted providers at VA clinics who attended a workshop on screening with training on improving communication with patients who had limited literacy skills. This technique resulted in increased screening recommendations to patients and increased screening completion rates

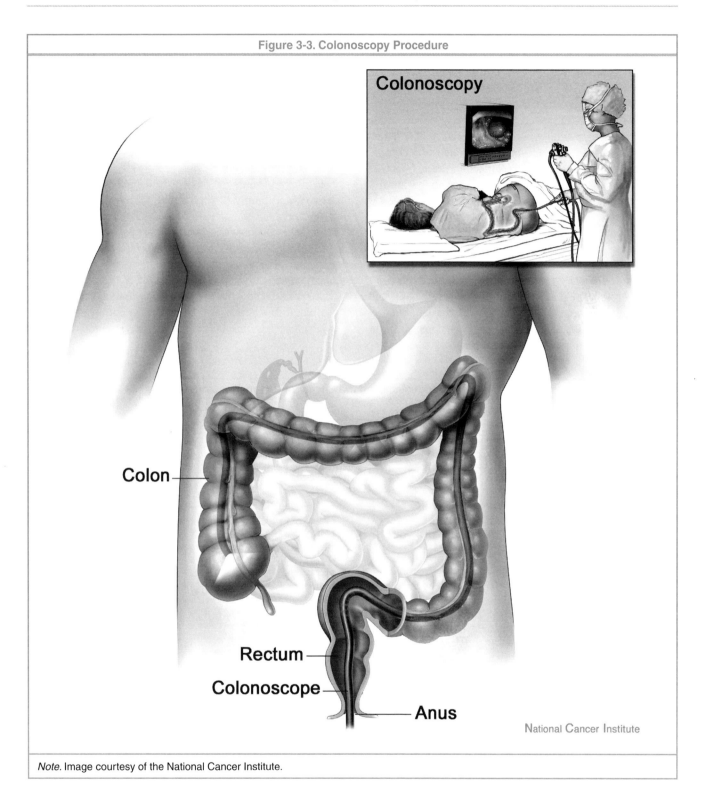

Figure 3-3. Colonoscopy Procedure

Colonoscopy

Colon

Rectum

Colonoscope

Anus

National Cancer Institute

Note. Image courtesy of the National Cancer Institute.

among veterans. In another study, FOBT kits were mailed randomly to selected people in the Midwest, some of whom received reminders to use them (Church et al., 2004). Direct mailing of the kits and reminders to participants increased usage of the kits.

Chemoprevention

Chemoprevention is the use of drugs or natural substances to inhibit carcinogenesis. Substantial epidemiologic evidence supports the view that chronic nonsteroidal anti-inflammatory drug (NSAID) use is associated with a reduced risk of developing several cancers, including colon and rectal. Aspirin and NSAIDs inhibit COX-2, which is expressed in 90% of sporadic colon cancers, and in adenomas of persons with FAP (Janne & Mayer, 2000). The evidence that NSAIDs reduce cancer risk is strongest for CRC. More than 20 studies have found a reduced incidence of CRCs or precancerous adenomas associated with chronic use of aspirin or other NSAIDs (Anderson, Umar, Viner, & Hawk, 2002). More than 14 published observational studies document the relationship between NSAID use and CRC incidence or mortality (DuBois, 2004). Figure 3-4 illustrates the development of colon cancer and the effect of NSAIDs on the process.

Two randomized controlled studies have shown the efficacy of aspirin in clinical intervention studies. Individuals with previously resected CRC, taking 325 mg of aspirin daily, had fewer adenomas recur compared to a placebo group (Sandler et al., 2003). In patients with a history of adenomas, aspirin

at a dose of 81 mg a day (not 325 mg a day) reduced adenoma incidence by 19% (Baron, Cole, & Sandler, 2003). Celecoxib, a COX-2 selective NSAID, also has been extensively studied. In addition to its role in FAP, it is being studied in the prevention of bladder cancer, regression of Barrett's esophagus, esophageal dysplasia, and basal cell cancers (Gordon, Kelloff, & Sigman, 2004).

Individuals who had used statins (pravastatin and simvastatin) for five years had a significantly reduced risk of CRC, even after adjusting for use of aspirin and NSAIDs, physical activity, and family history of CRC (Poynter et al., 2005). Folate supplementation (in multivitamins) has been shown to be protective against CRC after 15 years of use (Giovannucci et al., 1998). Calcium carbonate supplementation (1,200 mg of elemental calcium) in patients with a history of colorectal adenomas moderately reduced risk of adenoma recurrence (Baron et al., 1999). While these and other agents are being evaluated for their use in cancer prevention, randomized controlled trials must be conducted to confirm their value. In

Figure 3-4. Colon Carcinogenesis and the Effects of Chemopreventive Agents

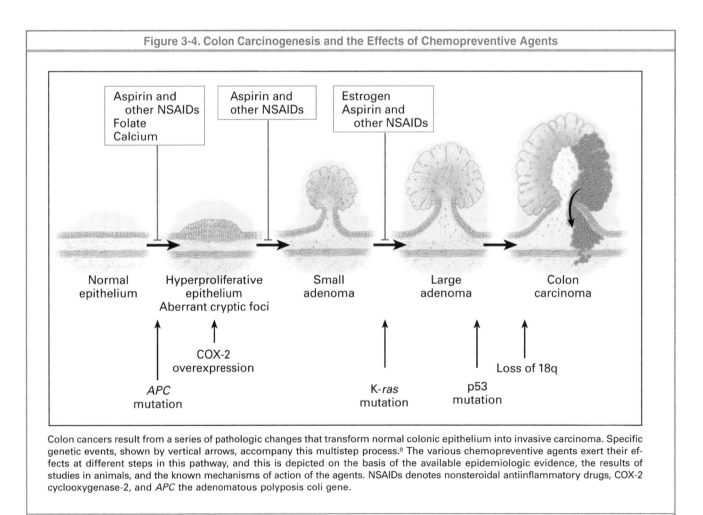

Colon cancers result from a series of pathologic changes that transform normal colonic epithelium into invasive carcinoma. Specific genetic events, shown by vertical arrows, accompany this multistep process.[8] The various chemopreventive agents exert their effects at different steps in this pathway, and this is depicted on the basis of the available epidemiologic evidence, the results of studies in animals, and the known mechanisms of action of the agents. NSAIDs denotes nonsteroidal antiinflammatory drugs, COX-2 cyclooxygenase-2, and APC the adenomatous polyposis coli gene.

Note. From "Chemoprevention of Colorectal Cancer," by P.A. Janne and R.J. Mayer, 2000, *New England Journal of Medicine, 342,* p. 1961. Copyright 2000 by the Massachusetts Medical Society. Reprinted with permission.

particular, potential side effects of aspirin and NSAIDs must be weighed against potential benefits.

Summary

The potential to prevent many GI cancers is great. Increasing amounts of evidence point to the prophylactic features of screening, and preventive measures in the form of NSAIDs are being studied. Modifying other risk factors such as obesity, diet composition, smoking, and alcohol intake also has the potential to decrease the incidence of these cancers.

References

Agrawal, S., Bhupinderjit, A., Bhutani, M., Boardman, L., Nguyen, C., Romero, Y., et al. (2005). Colorectal cancer in African Americans. *American Journal of Gastroenterology, 100,* 515–523.

American Cancer Society. (2005a). *Cancer facts and figures for African Americans, 2005–2006.* Atlanta, GA: Author

American Cancer Society. (2005b). *Colorectal cancer facts and figures, special edition.* Atlanta, GA: Author.

Anderson, W., Umar, A., Viner, J., & Hawk, E. (2002). The role of cyclooxygenase inhibitors in cancer prevention. *Current Pharmaceutical Design, 8,* 1035–1062.

Baron, J.A., Beach, M., Mandel, J.S., van Stolk, R.U., Haile, R.W., Sandler, R.S., et al. (1999). Calcium supplements for the prevention of colorectal adenomas. *New England Journal of Medicine, 340,* 101–107.

Baron, J.A., Cole, B.F., & Sandler, R.S. (2003). Randomized trial of aspirin to prevent colorectal adenomas in patients with previous colorectal cancer. *New England Journal of Medicine, 348,* 891–899.

Bond, J.H. (2000). Polyp guideline: Diagnosis, treatment, and surveillance for patients with colorectal polyps: Practice parameters committee of the American College of Gastroenterology. *American Journal of Gastroenterology, 95,* 3053–3063.

Chung, K.Y., Shia, J., Kemeny, N.E., Shah, M., Schwartz, G.K., Tse, A., et al. (2005). Cetuximab shows activity in colorectal cancer patients with tumors that do not express the epidermal growth factor receptor by immunohistochemistry. *Journal of Clinical Oncology, 23,* 1803–1810.

Church, T.R., Yeazel, M.W., Jones, R.M., Kochevar, L.K., Watt, G.D., Mongin, S.J., et al. (2004). A randomized trial of direct mailing of fecal occult blood tests to increase colorectal cancer screening. *Journal of the National Cancer Institute, 96,* 770–780.

Dannenberg, A., Lippman, S., Mann, J., Subbaramaiah, K., & DuBois, R. (2005). Cyclooxygenase-2 and epidermal growth factor receptor: Pharmacologic targets for chemoprevention. *Journal of Clinical Oncology, 23,* 254–266.

Dong, S., Traverso, G., Johnson, C., Geng, L., Favis, R., Boynton, K., et al. (2001). Detecting colorectal cancer in stool with use of multiple genetic targets. *Journal of the National Cancer Institute, 93,* 858–865.

Douglas, J., Gruber, S., Meister, K., Bonner, J., Watson, P., Krush, A., et al. (2005). History and molecular genetics of Lynch syndrome in family G: A century later. *JAMA, 294,* 2195–2202.

DuBois, R. (2004). Cyclooxygenase-2 inhibitors and colorectal cancer prevention. In G. Kelloff, E. Hawk, & C. Sigman (Eds.), *Cancer chemoprevention: Promising cancer chemoprevention agents* (Vol. 1, pp. 107–113). Totowa, NJ: Humana Press.

Enzinger, P., & Mayer, R. (2003). Esophageal cancer. *New England Journal of Medicine, 349,* 2241–2252.

Ferreira, M., Dolan, N., Fitzgibbon, M., Davis, T., Gorby, N., Ladewski, L., et al. (2005). Health care provider-directed intervention to increase colorectal cancer screening among veterans: Results of a randomized controlled trial. *New England Journal of Medicine, 23,* 1548–1554.

Garber, J., & Offit, K. (2005). Hereditary cancer predisposition syndromes. *Journal of Clinical Oncology, 23,* 276–292.

Giovannucci, E., Stampfer, M.J., Colditz, G.A., Hunter, D.J., Fuchs, C., Rosner, B.A., et al. (1998). Multivitamin use, folate, and colon cancer in women in the Nurses' Health Study. *Annals of Internal Medicine, 129,* 517–524.

Gordon, G., Kelloff, G., & Sigman, C. (2004). Anti-inflammatories and chemopreventional NSAIDs and other inhibitors. In G. Kelloff & E. Hawk (Eds.), *Cancer chemoprevention: Promising cancer chemopreventive agents* (Vol. 1, pp. 87–105). Totowa, NJ: Humana Press.

Herrinton, L.J., Selby, J.V., Friedman, G.D., Quesenberry, C.P., & Weiss, N.S. (1995). Case-control study of digital rectal screening in relation to mortality from cancer of the distal rectum. *American Journal of Epidemiology, 142,* 961–964.

Janne, P., & Mayer, R. (2000). Chemoprevention of colorectal cancer. *New England Journal of Medicine, 342,* 1960–1968.

Johnson, C., Harmsen, W., Wilson, L., Maccarty, R.L., Welch, T.J., Ilstrup, D.M., et al. (2003). Prospective blinded evaluation of computed tomographic colonography for screen detection of colorectal polyps. *Gastroenterology, 125,* 311–319.

Libutti, S., Saltz, L., Rustgi, A., & Tepper, J. (2005). Cancer of the colon. In V.T. DeVita, S. Hellman, & S. Rosenberg (Eds.), *Cancer: Principles and practice of oncology* (7th ed., pp. 1061–1109). Philadelphia: Lippincott Williams & Wilkins.

Lieberman, D.A., Harford, W.V., Ahnen, D.J., Provenzale, D., Sontag, S.J., Schnell, T.G., et al. (2001). One-time screening for colorectal cancer with combined fecal occult-blood testing and examination of the distal colon. *New England Journal of Medicine, 345,* 555–560.

Loescher, L., & Whitesell, L. (2003). The biology of cancer. In A.S. Tranin, A. Masny, & J. Jenkins (Eds.), *Genetics in oncology practice: Cancer risk assessment* (pp. 23–56). Pittsburgh, PA: Oncology Nursing Society.

Lynch, H.T., & de la Chapelle, A. (2003). Hereditary colorectal cancer. *New England Journal of Medicine, 348,* 919–932.

Macrae, F., & Young, G. (1999). Neoplastic and non-neoplastic polyps of the colon and rectum. In T. Yamada (Ed.), *Textbook of gastroenterology* (3rd ed., pp. 2023–2082). Philadelphia: Lippincott Williams & Wilkins.

Mahon, S. (2004). Colorectal cancer screening: A review of the evidence. *Clinical Journal of Oncology Nursing, 8,* 536–540.

Mandel, J., Bond, J.H., Church, T.R., Snover, D.C., Bradley, G., Schuman, L., et al. (1993). Reducing mortality from colorectal cancer by screening for fecal occult blood. *New England Journal of Medicine, 328,* 1365–1371.

Mandel, J., Church, T.R., Bond, J.H., Ederer, F., Geisser, M.S., Mongin, S.J., et al. (2000). The effect of fecal occult-blood screening on the incidence of colorectal cancer. *New England Journal of Medicine, 343,* 1603–1607.

Marshall, J. (1995). Technical proficiency of trainees performing colonoscopy: A learning curve. *Gastrointestinal Endoscopy, 42,* 287–291.

Merkle, C., & Loescher, L. (2005). Biology of cancer. In C.H. Yarbro, M.H. Frogge, & M. Goodman (Eds.), *Cancer nursing: Principles and practice* (6th ed., pp. 3–25). Sudbury, MA: Jones and Bartlett.

National Cancer Institute. (2005). *Colorectal cancer (PDQ®): Prevention, health professional version.* Retrieved March 1, 2005, from http://www.nci.nih.gov/cancertopics/pdq/treatment/colon/healthprofessional

National Human Genome Research Institute. (2005). *Hereditary colon cancers*. Retrieved June 1, 2005, from http://www.genome.gov

Pignone, M., Campbell, M., Carr, C., & Phillips, C. (2001). Meta-analysis of dietary restriction during fecal occult blood testing. *Effective Clinical Practice, 4*(4), 150–156.

Poon, R., Fan, S., & Wong, J. (2003). Clinical significance of angiogenesis in gastrointestinal cancers: A target for novel prognostic and therapeutic approaches. *Annals of Surgery, 238*(1), 9–28.

Porth, C. (2005). Disorders of gastrointestinal function. In C. Porth (Ed.), *Pathophysiology: Concepts of altered health states* (7th ed., pp. 885–915). Philadelphia: Lippincott Williams & Wilkins.

Poynter, J.N., Gruber, S.B., Higgins, P.D.R., Almog, R., Bonner, J.D., Rennert, H.S., et al. (2005). Statins and the risk of colorectal cancer. *New England Journal of Medicine, 352,* 2184–2192.

Reid, B. (2005). Barrett's esophagus. In G. Kelloff, E. Hawk, & C. Sigman (Eds.), *Cancer chemoprevention* (Vol. 2, pp. 325–342). Totowa, NJ: Humana Press.

Ribic, C.M., Sargent, D.J., Moore, M.J., Thibodeau, S.N., French, A.J., Goldberg, R.M., et al. (2003). Tumor microsatellite-instability status as a predictor of benefit from fluorouracil-based adjuvant chemotherapy for colon cancer. *New England Journal of Medicine, 349,* 247–257.

Rosen, A., & Schneider, E. (2004). Colorectal cancer screening disparities related to obesity and gender. *Journal of General Internal Medicine, 19,* 332–338.

Sandler, R.S., Halabi, S., Baron, J.A., Budinger, S., Paskett, E., Keresztes, R., et al. (2003). A randomized trial of aspirin to prevent colorectal adenomas in patients with previous colorectal cancer. *New England Journal of Medicine, 348,* 883–890.

Schmeler, K., Lynch, H., Chen, L., Munsell, M., Soliman, P., Clark, M., et al. (2006). Prophylactic surgery to reduce risk of gynecologic cancers in Lynch Syndrome. *New England Journal of Medicine, 354,* 261–269.

Steinbach, G., Lynch, P.M., Phillips, R.K.S., Wallace, M.H., Hawk, E., Gordon, G.B., et al. (2000). The effect of celecoxib, a cyclooxygenase-2 inhibitor, in familial adenomatous polyposis. *New England Journal of Medicine, 342,* 1946–1952.

Stucky-Marshall, L., & O'Brien, B. (2002). Gastrointestinal malignancies. In K. Jennings-Dozier & S. Mahon (Eds.), *Cancer prevention, detection, and control: A nursing perspective* (pp. 445–538). Pittsburgh, PA: Oncology Nursing Society.

Sweed, M., & Meropol, N. (2001). Assessment, diagnosis and staging. In D. Berg (Ed.), *Contemporary issues in colorectal cancer: A nursing perspective* (pp. 65–79). Sudbury, MA: Jones and Bartlett.

Takayama, T., Katsuki, S., Takahashi, Y., Ohi, M., Nojiri, S., Sakamaki, S., et al. (1998). Aberrant crypt foci of the colon as precursors of adenoma and cancer. *New England Journal of Medicine, 339,* 1277–1284.

Umar, A., Boland, C.R., Terdiman, J.P., Syngal, S., de la Chapelle, A., Ruschoff, J., et al. (2004). Revised Bethesda guidelines for hereditary nonpolyposis colorectal cancer (Lynch syndrome) and microsatellite instability. *Journal of the National Cancer Institute, 96,* 261–268.

Walsh, J.M.E., & Terdiman, J.P. (2003). Colorectal cancer screening: Scientific review. *JAMA, 289,* 1288–1296.

Wilkes, G. (2005). Colon, rectal, and anal cancers. In C.H. Yarbro, M.H. Frogge, & M. Goodman (Eds.), *Cancer nursing: Principles and practice* (6th ed., pp. 1155–1215). Sudbury, MA: Jones and Bartlett.

Winawer, S., Fletcher, R., Rex, D., Bond, J., Burt, R., Ferrucci, J., et al. (2003). Gastrointestinal consortium panel: Colorectal cancer screening and surveillance: Clinical guidelines and rationale-update based on new evidence. *Gastroenterology, 124,* 544–560.

Winawer, S., Stewart, E., Zauber, A., Bond, J.H., Ansel, H., Waye, J.D., et al. (2000). A comparison of colonoscopy and double-contrast barium enema for surveillance after polypectomy. *New England Journal of Medicine, 342,* 1766–1772.

Winawer, S.J., Zauber, A.G., Gerdes, H., O'Brien, M.J., Gottlieb, L.S., Sternberg, S.S., et al. (1996). Risk of colorectal cancer in the families of patients with adenomatous polyps. *New England Journal of Medicine, 334,* 82–87.

Winawer, S.J., Zauber, A.G., Ho, M., O'Brien, M.J., Gottlieb, L.S., Sternberg, S.S., et al. (1993). Prevention of colorectal cancer by colonoscopic polypectomy. The National Polyp Study Workgroup. *New England Journal of Medicine, 329,* 1977–1981.

Appendix A. Oncology Nursing Society Position on the Prevention and Early Detection of Cancer in the United States

In the United States, more than 1,280,000 new cancers are diagnosed in individuals across the life span each year. The lifetime risk of developing cancer in the United States is 43% for men and 38% for women. Cancer is the second leading cause of death in the United States, with one in every four deaths caused by cancer. Cancer is the leading cause of death in individuals 40–79 years of age (Jemal, Thomas, Murray, & Thun, 2002). Consequently, cancer is a major public health problem in the United States. Adopting healthier lifestyles and avoiding carcinogen exposure could prevent many cancers. According to the American Cancer Society (ACS), institution of prevention measures and early detection of cancer are two of the most important and effective strategies for reaching important public health goals of saving lives lost from cancer, diminishing suffering from cancer, and eliminating cancer as a major health problem.

It Is the Position of ONS That

Professional Education
- Oncology nurses, at both the generalist and advanced practice levels, must have educational preparation in the behavioral, biologic, educational, and economic principles of cancer prevention and early detection.
- Continuing education and specialized educational programs must be developed and provided to practicing nurses to facilitate integration of cancer prevention and early detection into clinical practice.
- Oncology specialty certification examinations and nursing licensure examinations should include evaluation of knowledge related to cancer prevention and detection practices in the general population.

Public Education
- All oncology nurses are well suited to provide education to the general public about prevention measures and general population screening guidelines for the early detection of cancer.
- Oncology nurses also are well suited to provide the necessary information and education to facilitate client decision making about participation in cancer prevention and control clinical trials.
- Oncology nurses must strive to provide comprehensive cancer prevention education and early detection services in a manner consistent with the cultural background and healthcare beliefs of individuals and families. Educational materials should be used that are targeted to the appropriate level of literacy and are culturally sensitive.
- Oncology nurses must be involved in the development of educational resources that have a focus on wellness, including the prevention and early detection of cancer in at-risk populations.
- Education programs must be developed and provided on the primary prevention of cancer (e.g., smoking cessation programs, nutritional counseling, avoidance of exposure to ultraviolet light) beginning in childhood and throughout the lifespan to encourage people to adopt healthy lifestyles.

Cancer Prevention and Detection Services
- Oncology nurses need to develop, implement, and evaluate measures to ensure that individuals and families have access to education about cancer prevention and appropriate cancer screening.
- Advance practice oncology nurses can obtain, document, and interpret cancer risk assessments; recommend appropriate cancer early detection and prevention strategies to individuals and families; and arrange or provide comprehensive cancer screening services based on the individual's level of risk. These practices must be consistent with guidelines defined by the appropriate state's nurse practice act, educational preparation, and role scope, along with standards of oncology nursing practice.
- As genetic technology evolves and knowledge of cancer genetics expands, healthcare providers must respond by informing patients, families, and the public about the implications of these developments for cancer prevention, early detection, and treatment. Nurses providing comprehensive cancer genetic counseling must be advanced practice oncology nurses with specialized education in hereditary cancer genetics.
- Individuals who have survived a cancer diagnosis also should receive age-appropriate cancer screening for other cancers.
- Programs that are focused on delivering services for the early detection of individual cancers (e.g., breast, prostate) also should ensure that patients receive education and are referred for screening for other common cancers. An immediate opportunity exists to implement this approach in men and women who are covered by Medicare and already eligible for reimbursement of the respective screening tests for breast, cervical, colorectal, and prostate cancers.
- Individuals should be assessed for eligibility for chemoprevention trials based on personal level of risk and referred for consideration at the appropriate clinical site.
- Individuals should be fully informed of their options for managing their personal risks for developing cancer and should understand the limitations, benefits, and risks of each strategy.

Research
- Oncology nurses need to conduct research to further assess the efficacy of cancer prevention and early detection programs, the psychological impact of cancer prevention and detection strategies, and promotion of participation in prevention and early detection activities.
- Research related to cancer prevention and detection strategies must be integrated into practice.

(Continued on next page)

Appendix A. Oncology Nursing Society Postion on Prevention and Early Detection of Cancer in the United States
(Continued)

Health Policy
- The development and evaluation of cancer prevention and detection health policy should be based on current cancer control research and involve multidisciplinary academicians and clinicians (including oncology nurses) and the public.
- Payors must be encouraged to provide coverage for prevention measures, counseling on prevention strategies, nutrition, and smoking cessation and for early detection and screening services based on individual risk levels.
- The ability to identify individuals who are at increased risk for developing cancer because of inherited altered (mutated) cancer predisposition genes is possible through cancer predisposition genetic testing. Risk assessment counseling and cancer predisposition genetic testing are components of comprehensive cancer care, and payors should cover them.
- Payors should cover clinical trials evaluating cancer prevention and detection strategies and chemoprevention.

Background
Primary cancer prevention refers to the prevention of cancer through health promotion and risk reduction. This includes carcinogen avoidance and, more recently, the use of chemoprevention agents and consideration of prophylactic surgeries in individuals at high risk for developing cancer, such as those with genetic predispositions. Secondary cancer prevention refers to the early detection and treatment of subclinical disease or early disease in people without signs or symptoms of cancer. Early detection is defined as the application of a test to detect a potential cancer in individuals who have no signs or symptoms of the cancer. Cancer screening refers to looking for cancer in a population at risk for a particular cancer. Cancer screening and early detection are forms of secondary cancer prevention aimed at detecting cancer early, when it is most treatable in asymptomatic people. Tertiary cancer prevention refers to the prevention and early detection of second primary cancers in individuals who have been diagnosed with cancer. This includes the application of specific tests to detect cancer and the use of chemoprevention agents to prevent the development of additional cancers.

Cancer continues to be a significant health problem in the United States. Everyone is at risk for developing cancer. Many cancers could be prevented by avoidance of carcinogens and mutagens. ACS estimated that 171,000 cancer deaths result annually from tobacco use and 19,000 deaths are related to excessive alcohol use (Jemal et al., 2002). An additional 185,000 cancer deaths are attributed to diet, nutrition, and other lifestyle factors and are probably preventable. Many of the 1.3 million skin cancers diagnosed annually could be prevented or controlled if people decreased their exposure to ultraviolet light. These facts underscore the importance of educating the public about the importance of a healthy lifestyle and strategies that can be instituted for the prevention of cancer. Public policy should support programs that provide education to the public about cancer prevention measures. Public education about the importance of cancer prevention measures and recommended cancer screening guidelines is an important component of oncology nursing practice and should occur both across the life span and the continuum of cancer care.

Cancer morbidity and mortality could be reduced further by the early detection of cancer in asymptomatic individuals. Cancers of the breast, colon, rectum, cervix, prostate, testis, oral cavity, and skin can be detected early, when treatment is more likely to be effective. These cancers alone account for about one half of all cancer cases diagnosed annually in the United States. ACS (2001) estimated that the current five-year relative survival rate for these cancers is about 80%. If all Americans participated in regular cancer screening, this rate could increase to 95%. Payors must include coverage of cancer screening services to achieve this goal.

Approved by the ONS Board of Directors, April 2001; revised August 2002.

The Board of Directors acknowledges the collective wisdom, contributions, and recommendations of these ONS members with recognized experience in the prevention and detection of cancer: Suzanne M. Mahon, RN, DNSc, AOCN®, assistant clinical professor in the Division of Hematology and Oncology at Saint Louis University in Missouri; and Lois J. Loescher, PhD, RN, cancer prevention fellow at Arizona Cancer Center at the University of Arizona in Tucson. The Board also acknowledges the contributions of Kathleen Jennings-Dozier, PhD, MPH, RN, CS, former associate professor at MCP Hahnemann University College of Nursing and Health Professions in Philadelphia, PA, who died from cancer in May 2002.

References
American Cancer Society. (2001). *Cancer facts and figures, 2001.* Atlanta, GA: Author.
Jemal, A., Thomas, A., Murray, T., & Thun, M. (2002). Cancer statistics, 2002. *CA: A Cancer Journal for Clinicians, 52,* 23–47.

Additional Resources
Carroll-Johnson, R.M. (Ed.). (2000). Cancer prevention and early detection: Oncology nursing's next frontier. *Oncology Nursing Forum, 27*(Suppl. 9), 1–61.
Jennings-Dozier, K., & Mahon, S.M. (Eds.). (2002). *Cancer prevention, detection, and control: A nursing perspective.* Pittsburgh, PA: Oncology Nursing Society.
National Cancer Institute, www.nci.nih.gov

CHAPTER 4

Esophageal and Gastric Cancers

Denise G. O'Dea, RN, NP, BC, OCN®, and
John S. Macdonald, MD

Introduction

Stomach

Stomach cancer represents a challenging problem in oncology. In 2006, an estimated 22,280 people in the United States will develop gastric cancer, and 11,430 will die of this disease (Jemal et al., 2006). Worldwide, 934,000 cases of stomach cancer are estimated to occur (Parkin, Bray, Ferlay, & Pisani, 2005), making this disease a major international cause of morbidity and mortality. In the United States, adenocarcinoma of the stomach was the most common cause of cancer-related deaths in 1900 and fell dramatically in the latter half of the century (Gunderson, Donohue, & Burch, 1995). The gastric cancer incidence rate of roughly 35 per 100,000 in 1930 fell to approximately 3 per 100,000 in the United States in the 1970s (Greenlee, Murray, Bolden, & Wingo, 2000). No adequate explanation is available for this change. It is of interest that the fall in gastric cancer incidence has occurred in the "endemic" or intestinal form (Boring, 1991) of the disease that usually is associated with preexisting intestinal metaplasia. This is the form of gastric cancer seen in high-incidence countries and appears to result from a combination of achlorhydria; migration of the small intestinal epithelium into the stomach, resulting in intestinal metaplasia; and superinfection with *Helicobacter (H.) pylori* (Parsonnet et al., 1991). This combination over time results in chronic gastritis with dysplastic changes and finally the development of the intestinal variant of adenocarcinoma of the stomach, the form of gastric cancer that has decreased significantly in incidence in the United States over the past 70 years.

A number of case-control epidemiologic studies have examined various factors associated with the development of the intestinal form of gastric cancer. Low socioeconomic class and low educational level have been associated with a higher incidence of gastric cancer. A higher incidence also has been shown in those who work in coal, nickel, and asbestos mining and in the processing of timber and rubber (Wu-Williams, Yu,

& Mack, 1990). Previous surgery for benign disease and, as noted previously, infection with the bacteria *H. pylori,* resulting in chronic gastritis, have been reported as risk factors for the development of gastric cancer (Parsonnet et al., 1991). It has been hypothesized that N-nitrosamine compounds act as carcinogens or cocarcinogens for the endemic form of gastric cancer. Positive associations seen in multiple studies have been diets rich in cured and smoked meats, salted fish, and bacon. Diets high in fruits and raw vegetables, fiber-rich bread, and increased amounts of vitamin C appear to provide some protection (Boring, 1991). The mechanism by which this protection is afforded is unknown but possibly related to the antioxidant properties of vitamin C and inhibition of N-nitrosamine formation. To date, convincing evidence of a strong positive association of the endocrine form of gastric cancer with smoking and alcohol intake has not been documented.

Esophageal

The American Cancer Society (2006) estimated that 14,500 new cases and 13,770 deaths from esophageal cancer will occur in the United States in 2006. Historically, the histology of the majority of esophageal cancers was squamous cell carcinoma. These tumors were located primarily in the upper or mid-esophagus. The main causative factors for squamous cell cancers have been identified as smoking, heavy alcohol intake, and diet, primarily a diet low in cruciferous and green and yellow fruits and vetetables.

Other risk factors for squamous cell carcinoma of the esophagus are celiac sprue, history of lye ingestion, and possibly hot liquid ingestion, which has been described in Chinese and South American populations. Human papillomavirus infection is being studied as a possible etiology. Squamous cell carcinoma is found more frequently in African Americans and Asians.

The incidence of esophageal cancer is increasing, but the most startling change in epidemiology of esophageal cancer is in histology. Adenocarcinoma of the esophagus is now more common than squamous cell carcinoma, especially in the United States and Europe. Since the 1970s, the incidence of esophageal adenocarcinoma in Caucasian men has increased yearly (Javle et al., 2006). Most tumors occur in the distal esophagus, gastroesophageal junction, and proximal cardia. Adenocarcinoma of the esophagus is associated with chronic reflux. Other risk factors are older age, Caucasian race, and obesity (Javle et al.; National Cancer Institute [NCI], 2006).

Gastroesophageal

Although the form of stomach cancer associated with *H. pylori* and chronic gastritis is decreasing, another type of gastroesophageal cancer has increased in incidence. These are tumors that do not occur on the background of intestinal metaplasia but develop in the gastroesophageal junction and distal esophagus and are cancers associated with Barrett's epithelium (gastric metaplasia of the esophagus) developing from chronic gastroesophageal reflux disease (GERD) (Macdonald, Hill, & Roberts, 1992; Wu-Williams et al., 1990). These tumors occur most commonly in middle-aged Caucasian males, and, although the distal esophagus is most commonly involved, the cardioesophageal junction also frequently exhibits tumor. It becomes difficult to determine whether these cancers are gastroesophageal junction stomach tumors or distal esophageal malignancies. The tumors associated with GERD also appear to be more common in obese men who drink alcohol and smoke cigarettes. It is considered possible that all three factors (drinking, smoking, and obesity) decrease the tone of the gastroesophageal sphincter mechanism and thus favor GERD (Macdonald et al., 1992). In many clinical trials and in clinical care guidelines, proximal gastric and distal esophageal cancers are treated in the same manner. Of note, the etiologic factors associated with the endemic form of gastric cancer and those resulting in distal esophageal and cardioesophageal junction neoplasms are very different. The endemic form of gastric adenocarcinoma occurs as a result of chronic gastritis with achlorhydria and *H. pylori* infection (Macdonald et al., 1992; Parsonnet et al., 1991). These etiologic factors may be assumed to be incompatible with, and actually may be protective against, tumors developing upon the background of Barrett's esophagus. Similarly, high gastric acid content and GERD are not compatible with achlorhydria, chronic gastritis, and *H. pylori* infection, and the development of the endemic form of gastric adenocarcinoma in such patients would be unlikely.

Diagnosis/Differential Diagnosis

Gastric Cancer

Initial diagnosis of gastric carcinoma often is delayed because patients are asymptomatic during early stages of stomach cancer. The symptoms of gastric carcinoma frequently are vague and nonspecific. They include complaints such as epigastric discomfort, nausea, vomiting, fatigue, weight loss, dysphagia, anorexia, regurgitation, early satiety, and eructation. Patients can present with gastric outlet obstruction as well as large bowel obstruction, depending on the location of tumor involvement. Dysphagia and symptoms of esophageal partial obstruction are increasingly more common because of the growing incidence of cardioesophageal junction tumors. Often the diagnosis is made in patients undergoing evaluation for iron-deficiency anemia and/or positive Hemoccult® (Beckman Coulter, Fullerton, CA) test. Patients with gastric cancer rarely present with significant bleeding. In the setting of acute upper intestinal bleeding, diagnosis of gastric leiomyosarcoma, gastrointestinal (GI) stromal tumors, or benign ulcer are more common than adenocarcinoma. In the United States, many patients with stomach cancer present with disease not curable by gastric resection. Commonly found physical findings in surgically incurable patients include palpable lymph node metastases in the left supraclavicular area (Virchow node) or left axilla (Irish node). Periumbilical nodules (Sister Mary Joseph node) represent peritoneal dissemination of tumor. Hepatomegaly or ascites may be present. Epigastric mass or pelvic masses due to Krukenberg tumor (ovarian metastases) or pelvic peritoneal drop metastases (Blumer shelf) may be detected on physical exam, and a careful pelvic/rectal exam should be part of the initial evaluation of all gastric cancer cases.

The double-contrast barium upper gastrointestinal (UGI) series still may be helpful in defining a gastric lesion (mucosa-based mass, ulcer, or peristaltic abnormality). However, now the most common diagnostic maneuver is upper endoscopy for direct visualization of stomach lesions, which can be biopsied for tissue diagnosis (Macdonald et al., 1992). In the case of submucosal tumors presenting as linitis plastica on UGI, blind biopsies may be helpful in establishing the diagnosis. Endoscopic ultrasound is useful in defining tumor penetration of the gastric wall (T stage) but is not as sensitive for detecting the presence of metastatic disease in perigastric lymph nodes. Diagnostic/therapeutic laparoscopy is useful in identifying cases with disseminated and/or technically unresectable disease and therefore may spare patients full laparotomy. The extent of disease at laparotomy usually is greater than predicted by pre-op evaluation. Computed tomography (CT) scanning and other imaging techniques provide additional information for staging purposes prior to laparotomy and assist in decision making regarding curative versus palliative resections. CT scanning, however, is an imperfect staging tool, having a reported accuracy rate ranging from 30%–72% (Macdonald et al., 1992). Understaging appears to be more of a problem than overstaging. Positron-emission tomography (PET)/CT scanning is being used frequently in patients receiving preoperative neoadjuvant therapy to indicate the possibility of disseminated cancers before curative resection is attempted. PET/CT also is being used to detect recurrent disease. The predictive value of this technology has yet to be defined. At the present time, no reliable serum tumor markers exist in gastric cancer. CEA and CA 19-9 have been noted to be elevated in approximately 40%–50% of patients with disseminated disease (Macdonald et al., 1992).

Esophageal Cancer

Esophageal cancer in the United States is most often adenocarcinoma but also can be squamous cell carcinoma. Adenocarcinoma most often afflicts Caucasian men, although an increase has occurred in the United States with African American men and Caucasian women. Lifestyle factors, such as obesity, GERD, and smoking, contribute to the growing rate (Ajani, 2005). Additionally, progression of Barrett's metaplasia to adenocarcinoma often is seen in the United States. Squamous cell carcinoma is associated with tobacco and alcohol consumption, poor nutrition, and low socioeconomic status (Ajani). Squamous cell is most common in endemic regions (see Figure 4-1). Screening of the population at large for esophageal cancer is not recommended, because it requires endoscopic intervention that is uncomfortable, requires sedation, and is not without risk. Complications of perforation, bleeding, myocardial infarction, and respiratory arrest have been reported at 0–13 per 10,000 procedures, with a mortality of 0–0.8 per 10,000 procedures (NCI, 2005). Endoscopies have been proposed every two to three years for people with Barrett's esophagus and no dysplasia (DeVault & Castell, 1999). For low-grade dysplasia, patients should have an endoscopy every six months for the first year and then annually; for high-grade dysplasia, patients may have surgical resection or serial endoscope evaluations (DeVault & Castell; NCI, 2005).

Diagnosis of esophageal cancer often occurs because of the symptom of dysphagia, and the patient may present with nutritional compromise and pain. Because of the ability of the esophagus to distend and the tendency of patients to modify their diets to alleviate the discomfort, dysphagia usually is a late symptom. Eighty to ninety percent of the esophagus may be occupied by tumor before dysphagia occurs (Javle et al., 2006). Patients then are diagnosed at the locally advanced or unresectable stages. The overall five-year survival rate in patients who are diagnosed at a treatable stage is 5%–30% (NCI, 2005).

Diagnostic staging tests are routine chest x-ray, upper endoscopy, CT of the chest, and abdomen and endoscopic ultrasound (EUS). EUS has 85%–90% accuracy in tumor staging. Other methods used include lymph node staging with fine-needle aspiration, thoracoscopy, and FDG (fluorodeoxyglucose) PET (NCI, 2005; Posner, Forastiere, & Minsky, 2005). There are no tumor markers in esophageal cancer.

Figure 4-1. Esophageal Cancer Staging

TNM Definitions

Primary tumor (T)
- TX: Primary tumor cannot be assessed
- T0: No evidence of primary tumor
- Tis: Carcinoma in situ
- T1: Tumor invades lamina propria or submucosa
- T2: Tumor invades muscularis propria
- T3: Tumor invades adventitia
- T4: Tumor invades adjacent structures

Regional lymph nodes (N)
- NX: Regional metastasis cannot be assessed
- N0: No regional lymph node metastasis
- N1: Regional lymph node metastasis

Distant metastasis (M)
- MX: Distant metastasis cannot be assessed
- M0: No distant metastasis
- M1: Distant metastasis
  Tumor of the lower thoracic esophagus
  – M1a: Metastasis in celiac lymph nodes
  – M1b: Other distant metastasis
  Tumors of the midthoracic esophagus
  – M1a: Not applicable
  – M1b: Nonregional lymph nodes and/or other distant metastasis
  Tumors of the upper thoracic esophagus
  – M1a: Metastasis in cervical nodes
  – M1b: Other distant metastasis

For tumors of the midthoracic esophagus, use only M1b because these tumors with metastases in nonregional lymph nodes have equally poor prognoses as do those with metastases in other distant sites.

AJCC stage groupings

Stage 0
- Tis, N0, M0

Stage I
- T1, N0, M0

Stage IIA
- T2, N0, M0
- T3, N0, M0

Stage IIB
- T1, N1, M0
- T2, N1, M0

Stage III
- T3, N1, M0
- T4, any N, M0

Stage IV
- Any T, any N, M1

Stage IVA
- Any T, any N, M1a

Stage IVB
- Any T, any N, M1b

Note. Data from *Esophageal Cancer Treatment*, by the National Cancer Institute, 2006. Retrieved March 30, 2006, from http://www.cancer.gov/cancertopics/pdq/treatment/esophageal/HealthProfessional/page3

Treatment

Surgery

The primary curative treatment of gastric carcinoma and distal esophageal cancer is surgical resection (Bonenkamp et al., 1999; Kodama, Sugimachi, Soejima, Matsusaka, & Inokuchi, 1981; Veverdis & Wanebo, 1992).

Gastric Cancer

In stomach cancer that is potentially resectable for cure (stages 0–IV M0), the surgical aim should be to perform a tumor resection entailing at least a partial gastrectomy with an *en bloc* (meaning in one piece as opposed to one node at a time) dissection of lymphatic tissue. For at least 20 years (Kodama et al., 1981; Veverdis & Wanebo, 1992), there has been an international debate regarding the most appropriate surgical procedures to use in cases of potentially curable gastric carcinoma. The point at issue is whether extensive *en bloc* lymph node dissection along with complete resection of the primary stomach tumor improves survival. The extent of resection is defined using a designation of D0, D1, and D2 (see Table 4-1). If a surgeon resects in an *en bloc* fashion, all of the tumor plus the N1 lymph nodes, a D1 dissection has been performed. If the N2 nodes are resected, this is a D2 dissection. If N1 nodes are not taken, a D0 procedure has been performed. The D2 dissection as a norm for gastric cancer surgery was developed from surgical practice in Japan. Japanese surgeons (Kodama et al.) for a number of years have reported superior results with the D2 surgical resection in gastric cancer. Small phase III comparisons of D1 and D2 dissections have been completed in South Africa and Hong Kong (Robertson et al., 1994). These studies were underpowered (less than 30 patients per arm) and showed no survival benefit for D2 nodal dissection. (Please see Figure 4-2 for staging definitions.)

Table 4-1. Gastric Cancer: Extent of Surgery

Resection	Definition
D0	Incomplete resection of N1 nodes
D1	Complete resection of N1 nodes
D2	Complete resection of N1 + N2 nodes

In the Netherlands, a much larger phase III study (Bonenkamp et al., 1999), including 711 evaluable cases, also tested D2 versus D1 dissection. This study demonstrated that the D2 dissection did not improve overall survival and was associated with a higher operative morbidity and mortality. This study also is of interest because it provided data for assessing the effect of extended lymph node dissection on staging accuracy.

A report by Bunt et al. (1995) demonstrated that patients undergoing D2 dissections had significantly more accurate surgical pathologic staging than patients undergoing D1 dissections. The Dutch investigators asked their pathologists to evaluate staging of patients under study who had undergone D2 resections. These pathologic specimens were first evaluated as if only D1 resection (removal of N1 nodes only) had been performed and a pathologic stage was applied. Subsequently, the whole specimen, including the N2 nodes, was evaluated, and the actual pathologic stage was defined (see Table 4-2). This study demonstrated that a D1 dissection, when compared to a D2 dissection, understaged 60%–75% of patients (see Table 4-2). For clinical scientists evaluating the effect of postoperative systemic therapy in gastric cancer, they should understand that less than D2 dissections result in a significant risk of understaging.

Irrespective of the surgical procedure used for treatment of gastric cancer, the effectiveness of surgical resection is poor. When survival of node-positive patients is examined after gastric resection in the United States, overall survival is, at best, 30% (Hermans et al., 1993; Macdonald et al., 1995). The development of symptomatic metastatic disease arising from unresected microscopic metastases present at the time of surgical resection is a cause of death. Because of the high risk of relapse after gastric resection, there has been a great deal of interest in strategies to prevent relapse and improve survival for patients with stomach cancer. The major approaches that have been explored have fallen into the categories of preoperative or neoadjuvant approaches and postoperative or adjuvant therapy strategies.

Esophageal Cancer

Early-stage esophageal cancers often are treated with endoscopic procedures, such as mucosal resection. This procedure may be curative in early cancers and can decrease the morbidity and mortality rates related to surgical procedures, such as radical esophagectomy. Careful patient selection is crucial in determining a treatment approach. Large randomized trials of early-stage esophageal cancers have not been conducted. Therefore, it is difficult to determine if surgical resection, endoscopic procedures, or chemoradiotherapy is the best approach (Urschel, 2006).

Early lesions in the esophagus can be treated with photodynamic therapy (PDT), laser treatment, and argon plasma coagulation, all of which destroy the mucosal layer of the esophagus with the goal of eliminating the premalignant cells. PDT, described in Chapter 6, is a technique where a photosensitizing agent, Photofrin® (Axcan Pharma, Birmingham, AL), is given intravenously to the patient 40–50 hours prior to use of a KTP laser during an esophagogastroduodenoscopy. PDT has shown some effectiveness in the treatment of high-grade dysplasia, but development of invasive cancers has been noted in 12 months during follow-up evaluations. Some authors recommended that PDT be offered only to patients

---

Figure 4-2. Stomach Cancer Staging

TNM Definitions

Primary tumor (T)
- TX: Primary tumor cannot be assessed
- T0: No evidence of primary tumor
- Tis: Carcinoma in situ; intraepithelial tumor without invasion of the lamina propria
- T1: Tumor invades lamina propria or submucosa
- T2: Tumor invades muscularis propria or subserosa*
  - T2a: Tumor invades muscularis propria
  - T2b: Tumor invades subserosa
- T3: Tumor penetrates serosa (visceral peritoneum) without invasion of adjacent structures
- T4: Tumor invades adjacent structure**, ***

* A tumor may penetrate the muscularis propria with extension into the gastrocolic or gastrohepatic ligaments, or into the greater or lesser omentum, without perforation of the visceral peritoneum covering these structures. In this case, the tumor is classified T2. If there is perforation of the visceral peritoneum covering the gastric ligaments or the omentum, the tumor should be classified T3.

** The adjacent structures of the stomach include the spleen, transverse colon, liver, diaphragm, pancreas, abdominal wall, adrenal gland, kidney, small intestine, and retroperitoneum.

*** Intramural extension to the duodenum or esophagus is classified by the depth of greatest invasion in any of these sites, including the stomach.

Regional lymph nodes (N)
- NX: Regional lymph node(s) cannot be assessed
- N0: No regional lymph node metastasis*
- N1: Metastasis in 1 to 6 regional lymph nodes
- N2: Metastasis in 7 to 15 regional lymph nodes
- N3: Metastasis in more than 15 regional lymph nodes

* A designation of pN0 should be used if all examined lymph nodes are negative, regardless of the total number removed and examined.

Distant metastasis (M)
- MX: Distant metastasis cannot be assessed
- M0: No distant metastasis
- M1: Distant metastasis

AJCC stage groupings

Stage 0
- Tis, N0, M0

Stage IA
- T1, N0, M0

Stage IB
- T1, N1, M0
- T2a, N0, M0
- T2b, N0, M0

Stage II
- T1, N2, M0
- T2a, N1, M0
- T2b, N1, M0
- T3, N0, M0

Stage IIIA
- T2a, N2, M0
- T2b, N2, M0
- T3, N1, M0
- T4, N0, M0

Stage IIIB
- T3, N2, M0

Stage IV
- T4, N1, M0
- T4, N2, M0
- T4, N3, M0
- T1, N3, M0
- T2, N3, M0
- T3, N3, M0
- Any T, any N, M1

Note. Data from *Stomach Cancer Treatment*, by the National Cancer Institute, 2006. Retrieved March 14, 2006, from http://www.cancer.gov/cancertopics/pdq/treatment/gastric/HealthProfessional/page3

Table 4-2. Gastric Cancer: Stage Migration: D1 Compared to D2 Gastrectomies						
D1 TNM		**D2 TNM**				
		Stage				
Stage	**Number of Patients**	**II**	**IIIA**	**IIIB**	**IV**	**% Change**
II	48	30	18			38%
IIIA	49		19	21	1	61%
IIIB	24			6	18	75%

Note. Based on information from Bunt et al., 1995.

who are not candidates for more extensive surgical treatments (Posner et al., 2005). To ablate or coagulate abnormal tissue, the neodymium yttrium aluminum garnet (Nd:YAG) laser may be used, which vaporizes tumor in order to palliate symptoms. Treatments are performed every other day for about a week and may be repeated every four to six weeks if symptoms

recur. Serious complications have been reported in 40% of patients (Javle et al., 2006). Endoscopic mucosal resections are an option for high-grade dysplasia or early neoplasms. This technique involves injection of fluid to float the lesion from the underlying layers, allowing greater resections.

Esophageal resection is the most effective treatment for cancers limited to the mucosa, but the most aggressive procedure, esophagectomy, is associated with substantial morbidity and mortality. Minimally invasive procedures, such as laparoscopic resections, are being performed in some centers, but long-term studies about patient outcomes are not yet available. Traditional surgical resections for cancer of the esophagus include the transhiatal esophagectomy, which involves a laparotomy and cervical anastomosis of the stomach to cervical esophagus after *en bloc* resection of the tumor; transthoracic or Ivor Lewis esophagogastrectomy, which involves a thoracotomy and laparotomy for anastomosis of the stomach to the cervical or upper thoracic esophagus and *en bloc* resection of the tumor; and left thoracotomy and left thoracoabdominal approaches (Posner et al., 2005) (see Figure 4-3). No significant differences in quality of life or survival

Figure 4-3. Total Esophagectomy With Gastric Anastomosis

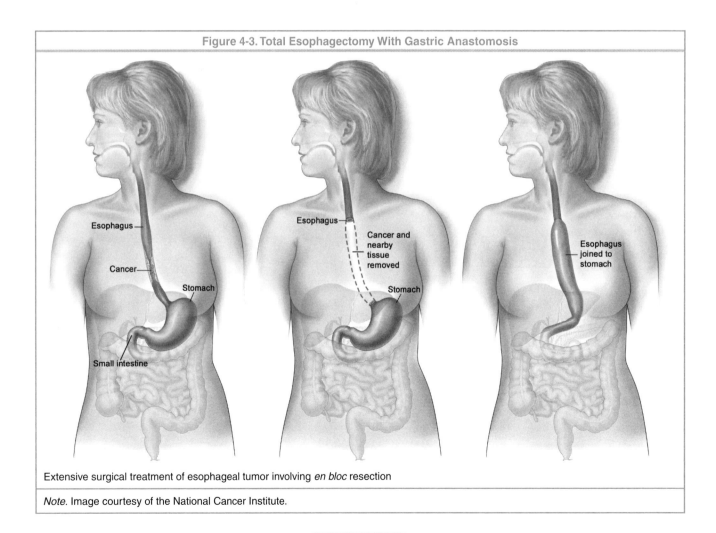

Extensive surgical treatment of esophageal tumor involving *en bloc* resection

Note. Image courtesy of the National Cancer Institute.

have been reported (NCI, 2006). Please see Chapter 6 for descriptions of the surgical procedures and management.

Adjuvant Therapy

Gastric Cancer

Adjuvant therapy of gastric cancer using systemic therapy alone or as part of combined modality therapy with curative intent also has been widely tested within the past three decades. Adjuvant cytotoxic chemotherapy alone has been of minimal benefit. Hermans et al. (1993) published a meta-analysis that demonstrated no conclusive value for adjuvant chemotherapy. Earle and Maroun (1999) published a meta-analysis that showed borderline statistical significance but clinically insignificant survival improvement from the use of adjuvant chemotherapy. In the United States, a clinical trial (Macdonald et al., 1995) testing 5-fluorouracil (5-FU), doxorubicin, and mitomycin-C (FAM) chemotherapy in a cooperative group (Southwest Oncology Group [SWOG]) also did not demonstrate any benefit for adjuvant chemotherapy. In this study, 191 patients were randomized between one year of FAM following surgery or surgery alone. No benefit from chemotherapy was observed, and the survival curves of treatment and control cases were overlapping. The overall survival at five years demonstrated in the study was approximately 35% for both surgery alone and for surgery followed by FAM chemotherapy. At present, adjuvant chemotherapy should be considered investigational. Newer regimens such as epirubicin, cisplatin, and 5-FU (ECF) and docetaxel, cisplatin, and 5-FU (DCF) have not been tested as pure adjuvant therapy in patients with resected gastric cancer.

One of the important therapeutic findings in gastric cancer over the past 15 years has been that in patients with known residual disease, the combination of radiation therapy plus fluorinated pyrimidine (5-FU) used as a radiation sensitizer could result in the complete control (apparent cure) of small amounts of residual or recurrent stomach cancer (Gastrointestinal Tumor Study Group, 1982). This use of combined modality radiation and chemotherapy also has been demonstrated to be efficacious in esophageal cancer (Herskovic et al., 1992) and has resulted, in that disease, in a prolonged disease-free survival of patients without the need for surgical resection. Because of the demonstrated benefit of combined radiation and fluorinated pyrimidine in patients with known residual gastric and esophageal carcinoma, a U.S. Intergroup study was initiated in 1991 to test whether the combination of 5-FU/leucovorin plus radiation therapy after surgical resection would be of value to patients with resected gastric carcinoma (see Figure 4-4). This study enrolled a total of 603 patients during a seven-year period of time and initially was reported in the spring of 2000 (oral communication, American Society of Clinical Oncology annual meeting) and was updated in September 2001 (Macdonald et al., 2001). This study included 281 eligible patients receiving 5-FU/leucovorin/radiation and 275 eligible patients in the observation arm. Eighty-five percent of cases in both arms had node-positive carcinoma (stage IIIA, IIIB, or IV). The types of surgery performed in this study were carefully analyzed. Results demonstrated that the standard of care in the United States does not include extended lymph node dissections. Fifty-four percent of cases underwent < D1 dissections (only partial removal of the N1 nodes), and only

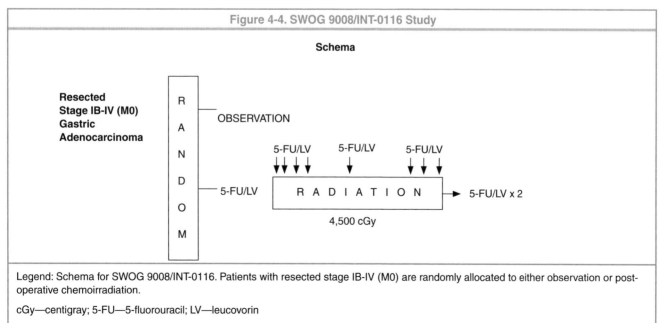

Figure 4-4. SWOG 9008/INT-0116 Study

Schema

Legend: Schema for SWOG 9008/INT-0116. Patients with resected stage IB-IV (M0) are randomly allocated to either observation or postoperative chemoirradiation.

cGy—centigray; 5-FU—5-fluorouracil; LV—leucovorin

Note. Based on information from Macdonald et al., 2001.

10% of patients were treated with D2 dissection (Macdonald et al., 2001).

Because the ultimate goal of adjuvant therapy is prevention of cancer recurrence and improvement in long-term survival, serious long-term toxicities of therapy are unacceptable. Combined modality therapy, as delivered in the phase III clinical trial (SWOG 9008/INT-0116), was well tolerated. Although 41% of patients experienced grade III toxicities and 32% experienced grade IV toxicities (mainly hematologic), only three patients (1%) died as a result of treatment (Macdonald et al., 2001). Careful review and verification of radiation treatment planning is necessary to safely and effectively deliver this combined modality therapy. When SWOG 9008/INT-0116 radiation treatment plans were reviewed before initiation of therapy, 34% were found to have major deviations. Two-thirds of these deviations would have resulted in undertreatment of patients, whereas one-third had the potential for delivering severely toxic radiation (Macdonald et al., 2001).

Combined modality 5-FU/leucovorin/radiation therapy significantly improved disease-free and overall survival (see Table 4-3). Median time to relapse was 30 months in the treatment arm versus 19 months in the control arm (p < 0.0001, two-sided P value). Overall survival also was improved, with a median survival of 35 months in the treatment arm versus 28 months in the control arm (p = 0.01, two-sided P value). Although there was a suggestion that combined modality therapy decreased local relapse (defined as relapse within the residual stomach), this was not statistically significant. The outcome data on SWOG 9008/INT-0116 were updated in January 2004 (Macdonald et al., 2004). At this time, median follow-up was seven years. Table 4-3 compares overall and disease-free survival outcomes from the 2001 and 2004 analyses. Results for the major endpoints of disease-free and overall survival did not change. The 2004 analysis confirms that chemoradiation results in prolonged and statistically significant benefit in disease-free and overall survival to patients with resected gastric cancer. These data demonstrate that the improvements in disease-free and overall survival do not

deteriorate over time. The 2004 analysis also shows that chemoradiation does not result in late toxic events leading to treatment-related morbidity or mortality in cases on the treatment arm. The significant improvements demonstrated in SWOG 9008/INT-0116 in disease-free and overall survival obtained with acceptable toxicity have made combined modality radiation chemotherapy a standard of care in patients with resected gastric cancer.

Esophageal Cancer

Surgery followed by chemotherapy is an acceptable treatment for many solid tumors, including breast and colon cancers. Unfortunately, this is not a very practical approach for esophageal cancer. Many patients take weeks to months to recover from esophagectomy. Clinical trials conducted in the past 10 years have not shown any benefit to postoperative therapy (Urschel, 2006). The chemotherapy agents used in these trials were platinum-based regimens. Current evidence does not support the routine use of postoperative chemotherapy after esophageal resection. Chemoradiotherapy after esophagectomy has not been studied in clinical trials (Urschel).

Although neoadjuvant chemoradiotherapy is the preferred treatment for esophageal cancer, adjuvant therapy is used in some situations. Palliation of symptoms such as dysphagia has been attempted with cisplatin (30 mg/m^2) and irinotecan (65 mg/m^2) weekly on days 1, 8, 15, and 22 followed by two weeks off and led to complete dysphagia relief in 70% of subjects (Ilson et al., 1999). Other trials have looked at paclitaxel and cisplatin, etoposide and cisplatin, and 5-FU and mitomycin C for dysphagia relief (Javle et al., 2006). The Eastern Cooperative Oncology Group evaluated adjuvant therapy of cisplatin (75 mg/m^2) and paclitaxel (175 mg/m^2) every three weeks for four cycles in patients with completely resected node-positive adenocarcinoma of the esophagus, gastroesophageal junction, or cardia and found that two-year survival was 60%, somewhat improved over historical controls (Kelsen et al., 1998).

Chemoradiotherapy, usually with cisplatin and infusional 5-FU, followed by esophageal surgery has been studied, with a resultant two-thirds of patients experiencing a downstage in their disease accompanied by survival advantage and improved local-regional control (Posner et al., 2005). The CALGB 9781 trial revealed that trimodality therapy was superior to surgery alone in stages I–III of esophageal cancer (Krasna et al., 2006). Trimodality therapy consists of cisplatin (100 mg/m^2) and 5-FU ($1,000 \text{ mg/m}^2/\text{day} \times 4 \text{ days}$) weeks 1 and 5 concurrent with radiation therapy, followed by esophagectomy. Results demonstrated a long-term survival advantage with the use of chemoradiation therapy followed by surgery; however, the trial consisted of only 56 patients, greatly limiting the study's generalizability. In metastatic disease, numerous agents have been used. Combination regimens of paclitaxel or irinotecan have higher response rates, but toxicities have been significant.

Table 4-3. SWOG 9008/INT-0116 Results		
	Chemoradiation	**Control**
Number of cases	281	275
Disease-free survival median (month)	30*	19
Overall survival median (month)	35**	28

* p < 0.0001
** p = 0.01

Note. Based on information from Macdonald et al., 2001, 2004.

Irinotecan and cisplatin may have the most favorable response and side-effect profile (Posner et al.).

Neoadjuvant Therapy

Gastric Cancer

Neoadjuvant treatment typically employs chemotherapy and/or radiation therapy before attempts of surgical resection of gastric cancer. Until recently, only phase II neoadjuvant studies have been reported. In spring 2003, the first well-powered phase III neoadjuvant chemotherapy study was presented at the American Society of Clinical Oncology meeting (Allum, Cunningham, & Weeden, 2003). The British Medical Research Council performed a clinical trial named MAGIC that randomly allocated 503 cases of potentially resectable gastric cancer to either preoperative or postoperative ECF chemotherapy versus surgery alone. Because of the general acceptance of postoperative chemoradiation as a result of the reporting of SWOG 9008/INT-0116, clinicians have been interested in comparing the outcomes of the MAGIC study with the results seen with postoperative chemoradiation. The results of the MAGIC study are illustrated in Table 4-4. Preoperative chemotherapy resulted in statistically significant improvement in disease-free survival. An increased rate of overall survival was seen at two years (48% versus 40%) with preoperative chemotherapy, but this improvement was not statistically significant. There was no excess in surgical complication rates for neoadjuvant cases versus surgery only cases. Toxicities with preoperative therapy were acceptable, and preoperative chemotherapy was delivered as planned in more than 91% of cases commencing chemotherapy. However, it was more difficult to deliver postoperative chemotherapy as planned, and only 133 (53%) cases commenced postoperative chemotherapy treatment (Allum et al.).

Two other important results were found in the MAGIC study. First, the curative resection rate appeared to be increased by neoadjuvant therapy. Surgeons were asked to assess whether a curative resection had been performed at the time of surgery. Operating surgeons estimated that 69%

of surgery-only cases were curatively resected versus 79% of patients receiving neoadjuvant therapy (p = 0.018) (see Table 4-5). Although the rate of curative resection was increased in the ECF-treated cases, the absolute number of cases resected

Table 4-5. MAGIC Trial Treatment Results: Effects of Neoadjuvant Therapy on Curative Resection and Downstaging of Tumors

	Epirubicin, Cisplatin, and 5-FU (ECF)	Surgery
Number of cases having surgery	212 (85%)	232 (92%)
Median time to surgery	99 days	14 days
Proportion of curative resections	79%*	69%*
Proportion T3/T4 tumor	49%	28%**

*p = 0.018
**p = 0.011

Note. Based on information from Allum et al., 2003.

in this arm was less (212 versus 232) than in the surgery-alone arm. This was because some of the patients randomized to neoadjuvant therapy never came to surgical resection. If the total number of cases randomized to the ECF arm is used as the denominator rather than those actually resected, the rate of curative resection would decrease in this arm. Although the increase in curative resection resulting from neoadjuvant therapy may be questionable, a significant downstaging of tumor occurred (surgery-only T3 = 64%, neoadjuvant therapy T3 = 49%, p = 0.011). In the results of the MAGIC study (tumor T stage) downstaging, some evidence of an increased rate of curative resection and increased disease-free survival clearly demonstrated that potentially important clinical benefits exist for neoadjuvant chemotherapy. However, it is not yet clear how neoadjuvant therapy may best be incorporated into the multimodality therapy of localized gastric cancer, particularly in regard to how this approach may be combined with postoperative chemoradiation (Allum et al., 2003).

In attempting to understand how neoadjuvant chemotherapy and postoperative chemoradiation may best be used in cases with resectable gastric cancer, clinicians have been interested in comparing the outcomes of MAGIC with those obtained in SWOG 9008/INT-0116. In attempting to compare MAGIC and SWOG 9008/INT-0116, it is helpful to compare patient characteristics (see Table 4-6). A similar number of patients are represented in both studies (> 500), with an equal frequency of T3/T4 tumors (approximately 65%) (Macdonald et al., 1995). The frequency of nodal metastases was greater in INT-0116 (85%) than in MAGIC (72%). Poor prognosis

Table 4-4. Result of Neoadjuvant Therapy: MAGIC Study Two-Year Survival

	Epirubicin, Cisplatin, and 5-FU (ECF)	Surgery Only
Progression-free survival	45%	30%*
Overall survival	48%	49%**

*p = 0.002 log rank
**p = 0.003 log rank

Note. Based on information from Allum et al., 2003.

Table 4-6. Patient Characteristics of INT-0116 and MAGIC Trials

	INT-0116	MAGIC
Number of cases	554	503
T3/T4	68%	64% (surgery only)
Nodes (-)	15%	28%
Nodes (+)	85%	72%
Nodes > 4	43%	27%

Note. Based on information from Macdonald et al., 1995.

cases with greater than four nodes involved with tumor were more common in INT-0116 (43%) than in MAGIC (27%). In general, the INT-0116 cases were at higher risk for recurrence than MAGIC cases. Although it is not possible to directly compare specific outcomes between the two studies using tests of statistical significance, it is possible to compare general outcomes (see Table 4-7). Cases treated with surgery alone did better in INT-0116 (52% two-year survival) when compared to the surgery-only arm of MAGIC (40% two-year survival). When the treatment arms were compared, two-year survival outcomes were better for INT-0116 (58%) than for MAGIC (48%). Validity for these general comparisons would need to be confirmed in prospective studies before any conclusions on relative efficacy may be drawn. However, because the MAGIC cases demonstrated that after preoperative chemotherapy, tumors were downstaged and resectability increased, both highly desirable results, and because INT-0116 demonstrated that postoperative chemoradiation increased disease-free and overall survival, one could argue that an important strategy in new studies would be to evaluate neoadjuvant therapy combined with postoperative chemoradiation. Such studies would require phase II pilot clinical trials to carefully assess patient tolerance of aggressive pre- and postoperative therapy. Combining neoadjuvant and postoperative chemoradiation may result in further improvement in outcomes for patients with resectable gastric cancer.

Esophageal Cancer

Two European trials conducted in 2002 and 2003 compared chemoradiation without surgery and neoadjuvant chemoradiation followed by planned surgery, respectively. A French trial (FFCD 9102) showed similar median survival in both groups. The chemoradiation group had a 19-month median survival and the chemoradiation plus surgery group was 17.7 months. Two-year survival was 34% in the neoadjuvant plus surgery arm and 40% in the chemoradiation arm. Ninety-day treatment-related mortality was 9% in the neoadjuvant surgery arm and 1% in the chemoradiation arm. But the surgical patients were less likely to need palliative endoscopic interventions (Urschel, 2006). The German Esophageal Cancer Study Group performed a similar trial that yielded similar results.

Berger et al. (2005) reported that complete response to neoadjuvant chemoradiotherapy in esophageal cancer is associated with improved survival. This trial of 171 patients with localized esophageal cancer received cisplatin-fluorouracil–based chemotherapy and a median radiation dose of 45 Gy (Berger et al.). A pathologic complete response was observed in 32% of patients, and some degree of response was observed in an additional 10%. The five-year overall survival rate was 26%, with a median survival of 33 months. For patients who achieved a pathologic complete response, the five-year overall survival rate was 48%, with a median survival of 50 months (Berger et al.). The authors of this study concluded that preoperative chemoradiation is not very effective.

The most recent findings suggested that chemoradiation followed by surgery prolongs survival (trial CALGB 9781) (Cintolo, 2006). This trial randomized 56 patients to receive chemoradiotherapy followed by surgery versus surgery alone. Follow-up at six years revealed a median overall survival of 4.5 years on the neoadjuvant chemoradiation plus surgery arm versus 1.8 years on the surgery-alone arm. Five-year overall survival rate was 39% for neoadjuvant chemo/radiotherapy plus surgery and 16% for surgery alone (Cintolo) (see Table 4-8).

Neoadjuvant chemoradiation therapy followed by surgery is an acceptable treatment option for a select group of patients.

Table 4-7. Two-Year Survival: INT-0116 and MAGIC Trials

Study	Surgery	Preoperative Chemotherapy and Postoperative Chemoradiation
INT-0116	52%	58%
MAGIC	40%	48%

Note. Based on information from Macdonald et al., 1995.

Table 4-8. Neoadjuvant Treatment of Esophageal Cancer: CALGB 9781 Study

	Trimodality	Surgery
Number of cases	30	26
Surgical complications	14	17
Deaths	0	2
Hospital days	11.5	10
Median survival (years)	4.5	1.8

Note. Based on information from Cintolo, 2006.

Large randomized trials are necessary to support the most recent findings of the CALGB 9781 trial.

Summary

What future approaches will be used in attempting to improve the survival of patients with stomach cancer? The results of SWOG 9008/INT-0116 demonstrated that for patients with gastric cancer undergoing gastrectomy in the United States, postoperative chemoradiation improves survival and future results in clinical trials. To be considered successful, patients must have outcomes equal to or superior to the treatment arm of SWOG 9008/INT-0116. The current National Intergroup Adjuvant Therapy Study (see Figure 4-5) for postgastrectomy cases tests ECF chemotherapy before and after chemoradiation compared to a standard arm, which is essentially the same as the treatment arm of SWOG 9008/INT-0116 (Macdonald et al., 2001). Another strategy of interest resulting from the recent evidence of benefit from neoadjuvant chemotherapy would be to combine neoadjuvant chemotherapy with postoperative chemoradiation. To fully understand the potential for combined modality approaches to gastric cancer management, clinical trials need to be mounted to critically evaluate adjuvant and neoadjuvant therapy strategies in appropriate groups of patients. For example, patients identified preoperatively should be candidates for phase III trials testing neoadjuvant therapy followed by surgery versus surgery alone. These preoperative cases also would be candidates for explanatory phase II trials testing the tolerability and efficacy of combined

pre- and postoperative combined modality therapy programs. Patients identified after gastric resection may be enrolled into the current U.S. Intergroup Study, which evaluates an improved chemoradiation regimen. The specific neoadjuvant and treatment programs of the future may use chemotherapy or chemotherapy plus radiation, as well as newer targeted therapies such as epidermal growth factor receptor (Cunningham et al., 2004) and/or vascular endothelial growth factor (Hurwitz et al., 2004) inhibition.

The treatment of choice for esophageal cancer remains surgery. Gastroesophageal tumors should be treated in the same fashion as gastric cancers. Future protocols need to be carried out to address the issue of targeted therapies in esophageal cancers, and therapies such as tyrosine kinase inhibitors and monoclonal antibodies may be of interest. Nurses must focus on educating the public about decreasing cigarette smoking and heavy alcohol consumption, because an increased incidence of esophageal cancers is associated with these risk factors.

References

Ajani, J. (2005). Carcinoma of the esophagus: Is biology screaming in my deaf ears? *Journal of Clinical Oncology, 23,* 4256–4258.

Allum, W., Cunningham, D., & Weeden, S. (2003). *Perioperative chemotherapy in operable gastric and lower oesophageal cancer: A randomized controlled trial (MAGIC trial) (249a).* Paper presented at the annual meeting of the American Society of Clinical Oncology, Orlando, FL.

Berger, C., Farma, J., Scott, W., Freedman, G., Weiner, L., Cheng, J., et al. (2005). Complete response to neoadjuvant chemoradiother-

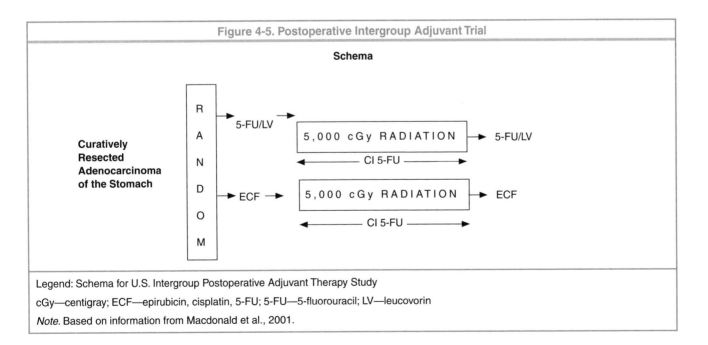

Figure 4-5. Postoperative Intergroup Adjuvant Trial

Schema

Curatively Resected Adenocarcinoma of the Stomach — RANDOM —

5-FU/LV → 5,000 cGy RADIATION → 5-FU/LV
← CI 5-FU →

ECF → 5,000 cGy RADIATION → ECF
← CI 5-FU →

Legend: Schema for U.S. Intergroup Postoperative Adjuvant Therapy Study

cGy—centigray; ECF—epirubicin, cisplatin, 5-FU; 5-FU—5-fluorouracil; LV—leucovorin

Note. Based on information from Macdonald et al., 2001.

apy in esophageal carcinoma is associated with significant improved survival. *Journal of Clinical Oncology, 23,* 4330–4337.

Bonenkamp, J., Hermans, J., Sasako, M., van de Velde, C.J., Welvaart, K., Songun, I., et al. (1999). Extended lymph node dissection for gastric cancer. *New England Journal of Medicine, 340,* 908–914.

Boring, H. (1991). Epidemiological research in stomach cancer: Progress over the last ten years. *Journal of Cancer Research and Clinical Oncology, 117*(2), 133–143.

Bunt, A., Hermans, J., Smit, V., van de Velde, C.J., Fleuren, G.J., & Bruijn, J.A. (1995). Surgical/pathological stage migration confounds comparison of gastric cancer survival rates between Japan and Western countries. *Journal of Clinical Oncology, 13,* 19–25.

Cintolo, R. (2006). Trimodality therapy effective in treating esophageal cancer. *Hematology/Oncology Today, 7,* 37.

Cunningham, D., Humblet, Y., Siena, S., Khayat, D., Bleiberg, H., Santoro, A., et al. (2004). Cetuximab monotherapy and cetuximab plus irinotecan in irinotecan-refractory metastatic colorectal cancer. *New England Journal of Medicine, 351,* 337–345.

DeVault, K., & Castell, D. (1999). Updated guidelines for the diagnosis and treatment of gastroesophageal reflux disease. The Practice Parameters Committee of the American College of Gastroenterology. *American Journal of Gastroenterology, 94,* 1434–1442.

Earle, C., & Maroun, J. (1999). Adjuvant chemotherapy after curative resection for gastric cancer in non-Asian patients; revisiting a meta-analysis of randomized trials. *European Journal of Cancer, 35,* 1059–1064.

Gastrointestinal Tumor Study Group. (1982). A comparison of combination chemotherapy and combined modality therapy for locally advanced gastric carcinoma. *Cancer, 49,* 1771–1777.

Greenlee, R., Murray, T., Bolden, S., & Wingo, P.A. (2000). Cancer statistics, 2000. *CA: A Cancer Journal for Clinicians, 50,* 7–33.

Gunderson, L., Donohue, J., & Burch, P. (1995). The stomach. In M. Abeloff, J. Armitage, A. Lichter, & E. Niederhuber (Eds.), *Clinical oncology* (pp. 1209–1241). New York: Churchill Livingstone.

Hermans, J., Bonenkamp, J., Boon, M., Bunt, A.M., Ohyama, S., Sasako, M., et al. (1993). Adjuvant therapy after curative resection for gastric cancer: Meta-analysis of randomized trials. *Journal of Clinical Oncology, 11,* 1441–1445.

Herskovic, A., Martz, K., Al-Sarraf, M., Leichman, L., Brindle, J., Vaitkevicius, V., et al. (1992). Combined chemotherapy and radiotherapy compared to radiotherapy alone in patients with cancer of the esophagus. *New England Journal of Medicine, 326,* 1593–1598.

Hurwitz, H., Fehrenbacher, L., Novotny, W., Cartwright, T., Hainsworth, J., Heim, W., et al. (2004). Bevacizumab plus irinotecan, fluorouracil, and leucovorin for metastatic colorectal cancer. *New England Journal of Medicine, 350,* 2335–2342.

Ilson, D., Saltz, L., Enzinger, P., Huang, Y., Kornblith, A., Gollub, M., et al. (1999). Phase II trial of weekly irinotecan plus cisplatin in advanced esophageal cancer. *Journal of Clinical Oncology, 17,* 3270–3275.

Javle, M., Ailawadhi, S., Yang, G., Nwogu, C., Schiff, M., & Nava, H. (2006). Palliation of malignant dysphagia in esophageal cancer: A literature based review. *Journal of Supportive Oncology, 4,* 365–373.

Jemal, A., Siegel, R., Ward, E., Murray, T., Xu, J., Smigal, C., et al. (2006). Cancer statistics, 2006. *CA: A Cancer Journal for Clinicians, 56,* 106–130.

Kelsen, D., Ginsberg, R., Pajak, T.F., Sheahan, D.G., Gunderson, L., Mortimer, J., et al. (1998). Chemotherapy followed by surgery compared with surgery alone for localized esophageal cancer. *New England Journal of Medicine, 339,* 1979–1984.

Kodama, Y., Sugimachi, K., Soejima, K., Matsusaka, T., & Inokuchi, K. (1981). Evaluation of extensive lymph node dissection for carcinoma of the stomach. *World Journal of Surgery, 5,* 241–248.

Krasna, M., Tepper, J., Niedzwiecki, D., Hollis, D., Reed, C., Goldberg, R., et al. (2006, January). *Trimodality therapy is superior to surgery alone in esophageal cancer: Results of CALGB 9781* [Abstract]. Paper presented at the American Society of Clinical Oncology Gastrointestinal Cancers Symposium, San Francisco, CA.

Macdonald, J., Fleming, T., Peterson, R., Berenberg, J.L., McClure, S., Chapman, R.A., et al. (1995). Adjuvant chemotherapy with 5-FU, Adriamycin and mitomycin-C (FAM) versus surgery alone for patients with locally advanced gastric adenocarcinoma: A Southwest Oncology Group study. *Annals of Surgical Oncology, 2,* 488–494.

Macdonald, J., Hill, M., & Roberts, I. (1992). Gastric cancer: Epidemiology, pathology, detection and staging. In J. Ahlgren & J. Macdonald (Eds.), *Gastrointestinal oncology* (pp. 151–158). Philadelphia: Lippincott.

Macdonald, J., Smalley, S., Benedetti, J., Estes, N., Haller, D., Ajani, J., et al. (2004). *Postoperative combined radiation and chemotherapy improves disease-free survival and overall survival in resected adenocarcinoma of the stomach and GE junction: Update of SWOG 9008.* San Francisco: American Society of Clinical Oncology.

Macdonald, J., Smalley, S., Benedetti, J., Hundahl, S.A., Estes, N.C., Stemmermann, G.N., et al. (2001). Chemoradiotherapy after surgery compared with surgery alone for adenocarcinoma of the stomach or gastroesophageal junction. *New England Journal of Medicine, 345,* 725–730.

National Cancer Institute. (2005). *Esophageal cancer (PDQ®) screening.* Retrieved September 28, 2006, from http://www.cancer.gov/cancertopics/pdq/screening/esophageal/

National Cancer Institute. (2006). *Esophageal cancer (PDQ®) treatment.* Retrieved September 28, 2006, from http://www.cancer.gov/cancertopics/pdq/treatment/esophageal/healthprofessional/allpages/

Parkin, D., Bray, F., Ferlay, J., & Pisani, P. (2005). Global cancer statistics, 2002. *CA: A Cancer Journal for Clinicians, 55,* 74–108.

Parsonnet, J., Friedman, G., Vandersteen, D., Chang, Y., Vogelman, J.H., Orentreich, N., et al. (1991). Helicobacter pylori infection and the risk of gastric carcinoma. *New England Journal of Medicine, 325,* 1127–1131.

Posner, M.C., Forastiere, A.A., & Minsky, D. (2005). Cancer of the gastrointestinal tract. In V.T. DeVita, S. Hellman, & S. Rosenberg (Eds.), Cancer: *Principles and practice of oncology* (7th ed., pp. 861–909). Philadelphia: Lippincott Williams & Wilkins.

Robertson, C., Chung, S., Woods, S., Griffin, S.M., Raimes, S.A., Lau, J.T., et al. (1994). A prospective randomized trial comparing R1 subtotal gastrectomy with R3 total gastrectomy for antral cancer. *Annals of Surgery, 220,* 176–182.

Urschel, J. (2006). Esophageal cancer. In A. Chang, P. Ganz, D. Hayes, T. Kinsella, H. Pass, J. Schiller, et al. (Eds.), *Oncology: An evidence-based approach* (pp. 664–679). New York: Springer.

Veverdis, M., & Wanebo, H. (1992). Gastric cancer: Surgical approach. In J. Ahlgren & J. Macdonald (Eds.), *Gastrointestinal oncology* (pp. 159–170). Philadelphia: Lippincott.

Wu-Williams, A., Yu, M., & Mack, T. (1990). Life-style, workplace, and stomach cancer by subsite in young men of Los Angeles County. *Cancer Research, 50,* 2569–2576.

CHAPTER 5

Colorectal and Anal Cancers

Joyce P. Griffin-Sobel, RN, PhD, AOCN®, APRN,BC

Introduction

Colon cancer is curable when diagnosed early, with a 90% five-year survival. Only about 37% of patients are diagnosed when the cancer is localized or confined to the adjacent nodes. With regional nodal involvement, survival is 25%–65%. With progression of the disease to metastatic sites, five-year survival decreases to 5%–7%. More than 50% of patients are diagnosed at stage III or IV (Meyerhardt & Mayer, 2005; Xiong & Ajani, 2004). With the advent of a large number of new chemotherapeutic and biologic agents, five-year survival in advanced disease is anticipated to increase. Recent data show that survival for patients with metastatic colorectal cancer (CRC) is now approaching 20 months with the use of the newer therapies (Kelly & Goldberg, 2005). Rectal cancer survival rates at five years range from 79% at stage I to 37% at stage III (Wilkes, 2005).

Characteristics

The colon and rectum make up the large bowel, or the portion of intestine from the ileocecal valve to the anus. It is divided into the cecum and appendix, ascending colon, transverse colon, descending colon, sigmoid colon, and rectum (see Figure 5-1). The rectum is the portion of the large bowel between the anal verge and the sigmoid colon, which extends from the anal verge to the rectal mucosa. The last 3–4 cm of the rectum is the anal canal. The wall of the intestine has four layers: serosa, muscularis, submucosa, and mucosa. Tumor penetration through these layers determines the stage and prognosis of colon cancer. New cells are produced in the crypts of Lieberkuhn, in the mucosal layer. Damage to these crypts can lead to the formation of adenomas (Takayama et al., 1998). Arterial supply to the colon is from the superior and inferior mesenteric arteries. The venous system drains into the portal circulation.

Histologic types of colon cancer include adenocarcinoma, the most common, subdivided into mucinous and signet ring adenocarcinomas; scirrhous tumors; and neuroendocrine

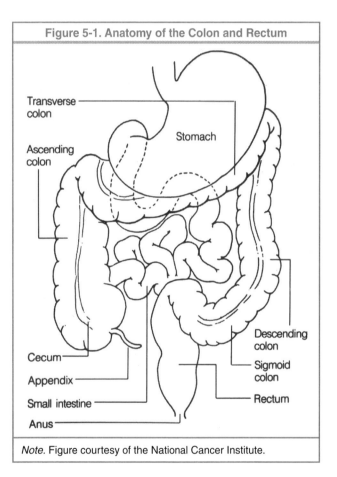

Figure 5-1. Anatomy of the Colon and Rectum

Transverse colon

Stomach

Ascending colon

Descending colon

Cecum

Sigmoid colon

Appendix

Small intestine

Rectum

Anus

Note. Figure courtesy of the National Cancer Institute.

tumors. Mucinous carcinomas are found in the descending colon and rectum and represent approximately 11%–17% of CRCs. Signet ring carcinomas, where intracellular mucin accumulation is noted, are rare, accounting for 1%–2%, and have a poor prognosis (Libutti, Saltz, Rustgi, & Tepper, 2005; Wilkes, 2005). Colon cancers are becoming more frequent in the proximal colon and typically are well differentiated but fungating. Tumors in the proximal colon account for 54% of colon cancers; 36% are in the descending or sigmoid colon; and 10% are in the transverse colon (Wilkes). Distal colon tumors in the descending and sigmoid sections of bowel may be more invasive. Metastases from the colon and rectum are most often to the liver and the lung.

The rectum is divided into three sections: the lower rectum 3–6 cm from the anal verge, the midrectum, and the upper rectum extending 8–10 cm from the anal verge (see Figure 5-2). Rectal tumors usually are described by their proximity to the anal sphincter musculature and anal verge. The mesorectum contains the blood supply and lymphatics for the rectum. A section of the rectum does not have a peritoneal layer, which may account for the higher risk of local recurrence than in colon cancer (Libutti, Tepper, Saltz, & Rustgi, 2005). Estimates for local recurrence range from 15%–45% after conventional surgery (Kapiteijn et al., 2001). Histology of most rectal cancers is the same as that of colon cancers: adenocarcinoma, which can be mucinous or signet ring. Carcinoid and neuroendocrine tumors also can occur. Preservation of continence and sexual function are primary goals of treatment whenever possible. Neoadjuvant therapy with radiation and chemotherapy can reduce tumor size substantially but does not negate the need for postoperative chemotherapy.

Carcinomas of the anal canal account for 1% of gastrointestinal (GI) cancers and usually are associated with infection by human papillomavirus (HPV), a sexually transmitted virus (National Comprehensive Cancer Network [NCCN], 2006a). In most cases, anal cancer can be cured with concurrent chemotherapy and radiotherapy. Rectal bleeding is the most common patient complaint, along with the sensation of a mass. A history of anal warts is present in 50% of homosexual men with anal cancer (Ryan, Compton, & Mayer, 2000). Women at a higher risk of developing anal tumors are those with a history of genital warts; infection with the herpes virus, chlamydia trachomatis, or gonorrhea; receptive anal intercourse; more than 10 sexual partners; and those with cervical, vulvar, or vaginal cancer (Ryan et al.). Patients who are HIV positive are two to six times as likely to have anal HPV, regardless of sexual habits, as those who are HIV negative and are twice as likely to progress to a higher grade of anal cancer (Ryan et al.). Tumor size is the most important factor in gauging prognosis, with lesions < 2 cm in diameter curable 80% of the time. Tumors greater than 5 cm are curable in less than 50% of patients. Squamous cell carcinoma (80%) and adenocarcinoma (15%) are the usual histologic types (NCCN, 2006a).

Diagnosis and Staging

A complete patient and family history should be obtained. Determine the presence of any significant risk factors, in-

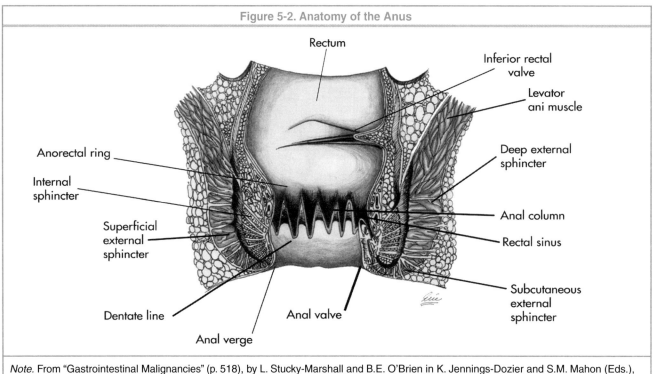

Figure 5-2. Anatomy of the Anus

Note. From "Gastrointestinal Malignancies" (p. 518), by L. Stucky-Marshall and B.E. O'Brien in K. Jennings-Dozier and S.M. Mahon (Eds.), *Cancer Prevention, Detection, and Control: A Nursing Perspective,* 2002, Pittsburgh, PA: Oncology Nursing Society. Copyright 2002 by the Oncology Nursing Society. Reprinted with permission.

cluding a history of inflammatory bowel disease, personal or familial polyps, or cancers. Assess for symptoms with a review of systems. Early CRCs present with few symptoms. Patients may complain of malaise, flatulence, and tenesmus. Tenesmus, or a feeling of incomplete evacuation, is a frequent symptom in rectal cancer. Patients may attribute blood on toilet tissue to hemorrhoids and regard it as an insignificant symptom unless specifically asked. As the disease progresses, patients may complain of blood in stools, change in bowel habits, abdominal pain, and cramping. Obstructive symptoms and weight loss may occur with advanced disease. Complaints of pain in the right side of the chest or abdomen may indicate liver involvement (Sweed & Meropol, 2001).

Physical examination findings may reveal a palpable mass, adenopathy, hepatomegaly, and blood in the rectum with left-sided colon cancers and rectal cancer. Melena may occur with right-sided tumors (Libutti, Saltz, et al., 2005). Sister Mary Joseph nodules, indicating a metastasis at the umbilicus, may occur in cancers of the stomach and colon (Sweed & Meropol, 2001). Auscultate for quality of bowel sounds before palpation of the abdomen. High-pitched sounds may be indicative of an obstructive lesion.

Complete blood counts and blood chemistries, including liver function tests, carcinoembryonic antigen (CEA), and coagulation assays, should be performed. Laboratory tests may be abnormal if metastases are present; liver function tests may be altered with liver metastases, or the patient may be anemic from chronic blood loss. Staging should include a colonoscopy and computed tomography (CT) scans. Positron-emission tomography scans, which highlight areas of high metabolic activity such as a tumor, may be performed to assess for liver and lung metastases. Endoscopic transrectal ultrasonography is indicated in staging of rectal cancers (Libutti, Saltz, et al., 2005; Libutti, Tepper, et al., 2005). Accurate staging helps to determine which patients may benefit from a local excision and which patients will require preoperative chemotherapy and radiotherapy to allow a tumor resection with negative margins. Anoscopy is recommended for staging of anal cancers.

Staging for CRC is done using the American Joint Committee on Cancer (AJCC) tumor, node, metastasis classification (Greene, Page, Fleming, & Fritz, 2002) (see Figure 5-3). Staging accounts for depth of invasion of the tumor into the bowel wall or surrounding organs and lymph node involvement (see Figure 5-4). AJCC and a National Cancer Institute (NCI) expert panel recommend that at least 12 lymph nodes be examined in patients with CRC to confirm the absence of nodal involvement (Greene, Page, et al., 2002; NCI, 2006). The number and size of nodes analyzed contribute to more accurate staging, especially in stage II cancer. One trial showed that five-year survival rates were significantly higher when at least 20 nodes were identified, compared with those who had less than 10 nodes examined (Le Voyer et al., 2003).

Figure 5-3. Colon Cancer Staging

TNM Definitions

Primary tumor (T)
- TX: Primary tumor cannot be assessed
- T0: No evidence of primary tumor
- Tis: Carcinoma in situ: intraepithelial tumor or invasion of the lamina propria*
- T1: Tumor invades submucosa
- T2: Tumor invades muscularis propria
- T3: Tumor invades through muscularis propria into the subserosa or into nonperitonealized pericolic or perirectal tissues
- T4: Tumor invades adjacent structures and/or perforates visceral peritoneum**,***

* This includes cancer cells confined within the glandular basement membrane (intraepithelial) or lamina propria (intramucosal) with no extension through the muscularis mucosae into the submucosa.

** Direct invasion in T4 includes invasion of other segments of the colorectum by way of the serosa; for example, invasion of the sigmoid colon by a carcinoma of the cecum.

*** Tumor that is adherent macroscopically to other organs or structures is classified T4. If no tumor is present in the adhesion microscopically, however, the classification should be pT3. The V and L substaging should be used to identify the presence or absence of vascular or lymphatic invasion.

Regional lymph nodes (N)
- NX: Regional lymph node(s) cannot be assessed
- N0: No regional lymph node metastasis
- N1: Metastasis in 1 to 3 regional lymph nodes
- N2: Metastasis in 4 or more regional lymph nodes

Distant metastasis (M)
- MX: Distant metastasis cannot be assessed
- M0: No distant metastasis
- M1: Distant metastasis

AJCC stage groupings

Stage 0
- Tis, N0, M0

Stage I
- T1, N0, M0
- T2, N0, M0

Stage IIA
- T3, N0, M0

Stage IIB
- T4, N0, M0

Stage IIIA
- T1, N1, M0
- T2, N1, M0

Stage IIIB
- T3, N1, M0
- T4, N1, M0

Stage IIIC
- Any T, N2, M0

Stage IV
- Any T, any N, M1

Note. Data from *Colon Cancer Treatment*, by the National Cancer Institute, 2006. Retrieved March 15, 2006, from http://www.cancer.gov/cancertopics/pdq/treatment/colon/HealthProfessional/page3

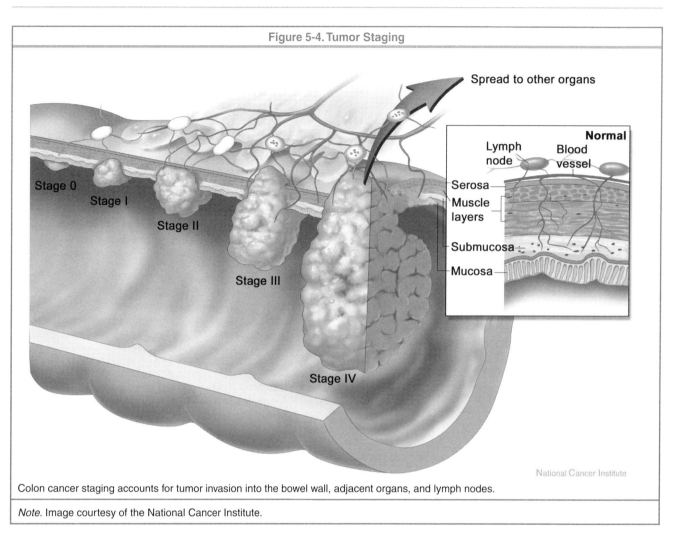

Figure 5-4. Tumor Staging

Spread to other organs

Stage 0

Stage I

Stage II

Stage III

Stage IV

Normal

Lymph node

Blood vessel

Serosa

Muscle layers

Submucosa

Mucosa

National Cancer Institute

Colon cancer staging accounts for tumor invasion into the bowel wall, adjacent organs, and lymph nodes.

Note. Image courtesy of the National Cancer Institute.

Prognostic Factors

For patients with N0 or N1 disease (one to three positive lymph nodes), patients with T1 or T2 disease have a significantly better prognosis than those with larger tumors (T3 or T4). When patients have four or more positive nodes, the prognosis is poor despite the T stage. Therefore, stages IIIA, IIIB, and IIIC have significant prognostic value, with stage IIIA at 59.8%, stage IIIB at 42%, and stage IIIC at 27.3% for five-year survival (Greene, Stewart, & Norton, 2002; Meyerhardt & Mayer, 2005). Additionally, tumors that are completely resected, leaving negative surgical margins, imply a better prognosis than those that leave microscopically or grossly positive margins. Patients with elevated CEA levels (greater than 5 mg/ml) preoperatively and patients whose CEA does not normalize postoperatively have a higher risk of recurrence (Libutti, Saltz, et al., 2005; Wolmark et al., 1984).

Surgical Management

Surgery is the primary treatment for most CRCs and offers the greatest potential for cure. The NCCN (2006b) guidelines for colon cancer recommend a colectomy with removal of regional lymph nodes and associated blood vessels for resectable colon cancers. Location, size, and degree of invasiveness of the tumor determine the type of surgery performed. The patient's overall physical condition also is part of the decision. Surgical procedures for cancer of the colon include

- Resection with anastomosis, in which the tumor is removed along with a segment of bowel, regional lymph nodes, and blood vessels (see Figure 5-5). Laparoscopic techniques may be used.
- Hemicolectomy, either right or left. Right hemicolectomy involves removal of the bowel from the distal ileum to the middle of the transverse colon, whereas left involves removal from mid-transverse colon up to and including the rectum.
- Abdominoperineal resection with permanent sigmoid colostomy, which includes removal of the sigmoid colon and rectum. This procedure involves abdominal and perianal incisions because the bowel is dissected free of associated structures transabdominally and removed in a perineal resection.

Figure 5-5. Resection With Anastomosis

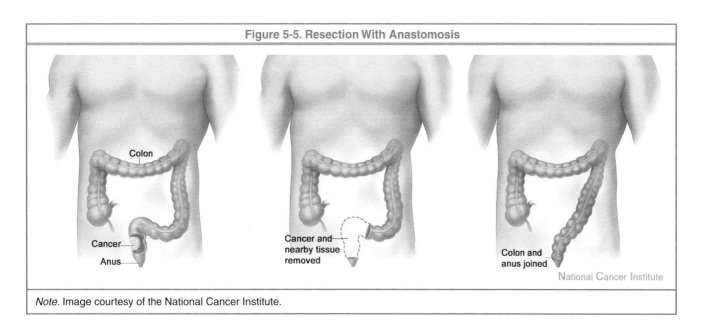

Note. Image courtesy of the National Cancer Institute.

- Lower anterior resections, primarily for tumors of the rectum. This involves removal of distal descending colon, sigmoid, and upper rectum (see Figure 5-6). Neoadjuvant chemotherapy and radiotherapy techniques increasingly are being used to shrink tumor size preoperatively and avoid loss of anal sphincters and need for ostomies.
- Temporary colostomies, which are performed to allow initial bowel decompression with subsequent resection (Manning, 2004; Wilkes, 2005).

Patients who require an ostomy should be seen by an enterostomal therapy nurse (certified in wound, ostomy, and continence nursing) preoperatively to ensure that the stoma is placed in the correct place on the abdominal wall. Incorrect placement may interfere with clothing or belt placement, resulting in inconvenience for the patient. If the stoma is placed in a skin fold, the stoma bag may not remain in place. Preoperative teaching is essential to aid the patient in coping with a stoma and allowing the patient to verbalize concerns about body image and sexuality during adaptation. Many communities have ostomy clubs, and someone who has been successfully living with an ostomy can visit the patient and provide support.

Laparoscopic colectomy has become increasingly common for management of early-stage tumors. The perceived advantages of less postoperative recovery time, decreased pain, and reduced length of stay that is associated with a laparoscopic resection must be balanced with the inability of the surgeon

---

Figure 5-6. Anterior Resection

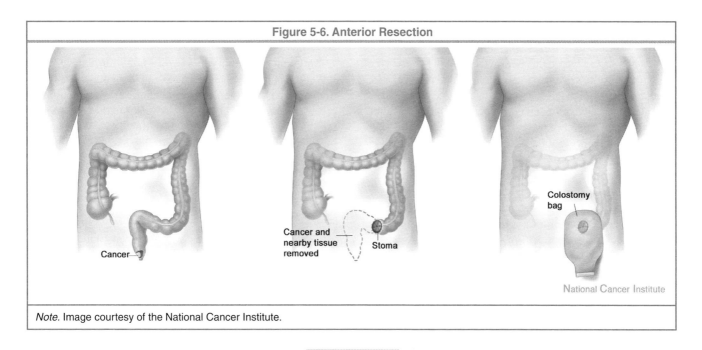

Note. Image courtesy of the National Cancer Institute.

---

to explore the surgical area thoroughly with this approach. Randomized controlled studies have compared laparoscopic resection for colon cancer with traditional surgical techniques and have reported similar outcomes in recurrence rates and overall survival at three years (Clinical Outcomes of Surgical Therapy Study Group, 2004). Operating room time was longer but hospital stay was shorter for the laparoscopic patients (Rossi & Rothenberger, 2006). NCCN (2006b) guidelines state that laparoscopic colectomy may be considered if the surgeon is experienced in this operative technique and the disease is not locally advanced or metastatic. Thorough abdominal exploration is required.

Colon tumors most frequently metastasize to the liver and lungs. Surgical resection is curative in 25%–40% of patients with resectable liver metastases (NCI, 2006). Surgical resection of hepatic metastases is increasingly common in carefully selected patients, with five-year survival close to 60%; however, most cases are inoperable because of number, size, or location of the metastases (Bilchik et al., 2005). When liver disease is initially unresectable, neoadjuvant chemotherapy may be prescribed. Studies have reported use of IFL (irinotecan, 5-fluorouracil [5-FU], and leucovorin [LV]) or FOLFOX4 (oxaliplatin, 5-FU, and LV) with 32.5%–41% of patients able to have subsequent resections (Alberts et al., 2003; Pozzo et al., 2004). Improvements in systemic therapy may increase the number of patients with resectable metastases. Adjuvant chemotherapy should follow resection of metastases. Ablative therapy to the liver using radiofrequency ablation or cryosurgery also can be performed (NCCN, 2006b).

Reports have emerged of liver complications in patients treated with chemotherapy, particularly oxaliplatin. These complications include vascular changes or blue liver syndrome, which consists of a blue discoloration and an edematous, spongy liver accompanied by a decrease in liver function capacity. Other noted abnormalities include hepatic sinusoidal abnormalities, similar to veno-occlusive disease, and steatohepatitis, or fatty liver disease (Bilchik et al., 2005).

Rectal cancers may be treated with sphincter-preserving transanal excision, low anterior resection, or abdominoperineal resection. Endorectal ultrasound or pelvic magnetic resonance imaging (MRI) allows the surgeon to evaluate the layers of the rectal wall and depth of invasion (Greene, Page, et al., 2002). The type of surgery recommended is made based on depth of invasiveness into the muscle wall, the location of the lesion in relation to the anal verge, and the appearance of the cancer.

The latest NCCN guidelines for rectal cancer (2006c) made the following surgical recommendations.
- Transanal excisions for tumors within 8 cm of the anal verge, < 3 cm size or < 30% of the bowel circumference
- Transabdominal (abdominoperineal, lower anterior, or coloanal anastomoses using mesorectal excisions) for tumors not amenable to local surgical techniques
- Biopsy or removal of clinically suspicious nodes beyond the resection area

The local recurrence rate after transanal excision has been reported to be 25% (Sengupta & Tjandra, 2001). To decrease that recurrence rate, NCCN (2006c) recommended a transabdominal resection if tumor margins are not clear or the tumor is not well differentiated. Lesions in the lower rectum often require abdominoperineal resections or colo-anal anastomosis, with a mesorectal excision to decrease recurrence rates. Abdominoperineal resections, with placement of a colostomy, are the traditional surgery for patients with tumors in the distal rectum. However, newer surgical techniques such as creation of end-to-end anastomoses allow preservation of the anal sphincter (Nelson et al., 2001). Adjuvant radiotherapy and chemotherapy should be given, either pre- or postoperatively, to patients with lymph node–negative T3 or T4 lesions and any lymph node–positive cancer. Radiation is given to decrease the incidence of local recurrences, which range from 25%–50% in patients with node-positive T3/T4 disease (Libutti, Tepper, et al., 2005). A definitive study on this treatment was conducted in Sweden, where 1,861 patients with resectable rectal cancer were randomized to preoperative radiotherapy followed by total mesorectal excision or to mesorectal excision alone. Survival at two years was equivalent; however, local recurrence was 8.2% in the surgery arm and 2.4% (p < 0.001) in the radiation and surgery arm (Kapiteijn et al., 2001). Local and regional recurrence is further decreased by the use of concurrent chemotherapy.

NCCN guidelines for anal cancer recommended local excision with adequate margins, followed by radiation therapy and chemotherapy with mitomycin and 5-FU (NCCN, 2006a). For patients with T1/T2, N0 lesions, the radiation dose should be 45–59 Gray (Gy), and larger lesions should receive 55–59 Gy. The field should include both the inguinal and pelvic nodes. Randomized clinical trials support the efficacy of this treatment with a lower subsequent colostomy rate and higher disease-free survival in patients who received the combination chemoradiation (NCCN, 2006a).

Surgical complications include infection, anastomotic leak, bleeding, wound dehiscence, and impaired bowel function. Adequate preoperative bowel preparation is essential for preventing wound and intra-abdominal infections. Mobilizing the patient as soon as possible after surgery will help to prevent complications from immobility such as thromboses and pneumonia.

Chemotherapeutic Management

Significant advancements in the treatment of localized and advanced CRC have occurred in the past decade. Four-year overall survival is now approaching 80% (Allegra & Sargent, 2005; Andre, Boni, et al., 2004). Older adults also benefit significantly from adjuvant chemotherapy, and it should be routinely offered to them (Sargent et al., 2001).

Colon Cancer

The stage of the cancer determines the need for additional treatment after surgery. For those with stage III disease, adjuvant treatment is recommended, which decreases the risk of death by one-third when compared to surgery alone (Laurie et al., 1989; Moertel et al., 1990). Using adjuvant chemotherapy routinely for stage II patients is controversial, unless the patient is at high risk. The American Society of Clinical Oncology concluded that adjuvant chemotherapy should not be used routinely for patients with stage II disease unless they are at high risk for recurrence (Benson et al., 2004). However, a more recent study showed a small (3%–4%) but statistically significant benefit for adjuvant treatment with 5-FU/LV over observation alone. Five-year survival rate with 5-FU/LV was 80.3%, compared to 77% in the control arm (Gray et al., 2004). For patients with metastatic disease, chemotherapy has improved one-year survival from 34% to 50% (Meyerhardt & Mayer, 2005).

5-Fluorouracil

The mainstay of therapy for CRC for many years has been 5-FU, initially with levamisole, which later was replaced with LV. 5-FU acts by inhibiting thymidylate synthase. Levamisole was used because it was thought to be an immune modulator when used with 5-FU (Moertel et al., 1995). It has no impact on survival when used alone (Andre, de Gramont, Study Group of Clinical Research in Radiotherapies Oncology, & Oncology Multidiciplinary Research Group, 2004). However, LV, which enhances the activity of 5-FU by inhibiting DNA synthesis by slowing its degradation, has largely replaced levamisole in therapy. It was demonstrated that six months of 5-FU with LV was at least as active as 12 months of 5-FU with levamisole (Moertel et al., 1995). This study made six months of 5-FU/LV the standard adjuvant therapy for stage III cancer. A large number of studies have examined 5-FU in various permutations of administration: bolus, infusional, with levamisole, and with LV. All methods of 5-FU administration (weekly, monthly, bolus, biweekly, infusional, and oral) are similarly effective (Kelly & Goldberg, 2005) (see Figure 5-7). Survival advantages have been demonstrated with bolus IV 5-FU plus LV administered according to the Mayo Clinic regimen (five days, monthly, six months) or the Roswell Park regimen (weekly bolus, six of every eight weeks, eight months) (Haller et al., 1998). However, the most recent data show that infusional regimens of 5-FU/LV are safer than bolus regimens because of reduced toxicity (Sun & Haller, 2005). A trial that directly compared infusional administration to the bolus method (Mayo Clinic regimen) demonstrated no difference in efficacy, but fewer side effects, including diarrhea, neutropenia, and mucositis, were reported with the infusional regimen (Andre et al., 2003).

The benefits of 5-FU–based adjuvant chemotherapy in reducing the risk of relapse and prolonging survival in patients with resected colon cancer are well established in

---

Figure 5-7. Chemotherapeutic Treatments for Colon Cancer

U.S. Food and Drug Administration (FDA)–approved agents
- Fluorouracil (5-FU)
- Capecitabine (Xeloda®)
- Irinotecan (Camptosar®)
- Oxaliplatin (Eloxatin®)
- Cetuximab (Erbitux®)
- Bevacizumab (Avastin®)

FDA-approved regimens
- 5-FU
  - Mayo Clinic regimen—leucovorin (LV) 20 mg/m² IV bolus days 1–5; 5-FU 425 mg/m² IV bolus days 1–5, repeat every 4–5 weeks x 6 cycles
  - Roswell Park regimen—LV 500 mg/m² IV over 2 hours; 5-FU 500 mg/m² IV bolus days 1, 8, 15, 22, 29, 36, repeat every 6–8 weeks x 4 cycles
  - de Gramont regimen—LV 400 mg/m² IV days 1 and 2; 5-FU 400 mg/m² IV bolus; 600 mg/m²; 5-FU continuous infusion, days 1–2; repeat every 2 weeks
- Capecitabine 1,250 mg/m² po twice daily days 1–14 every 3 weeks x 24 weeks
- IFL—Irinotecan, bolus 5-FU, and LV
  - On days 1, 8, 15, 22—Irinotecan 125 mg/m² IV over 90 minutes, LV 20 mg/m² IV bolus, 5-FU 500 mg/m² IV bolus, days 1, 8, 15, 22; repeat every 6 weeks; approved for first-line therapy
- Irinotecan 125 mg/m² IV over 30–90 minutes, days 1, 8, 15, 22; repeat every 6 weeks
- FOLFIRI—Irinotecan, 5-FU, and LV
  - On day 1—Irinotecan 180 mg/m² IV over 2 hours; LV 400 mg/m² IV over 2 hours prior to 5-FU on days 1 and 2; 5-FU 400 mg/m² IV bolus days 1 and 2
  - On days 1 and 2—Continuous-infusion 5-FU 600 mg/m² for 22 hours; repeat every 2 weeks; approved first-line therapy
- FOLFOX4—Oxaliplatin, 5-FU, and LV
  - On day 1—Oxaliplatin 85 mg/m² IV over 2 hours
  - On days 1 and 2—LV 200 mg/m² IV over 2 hours; 5-FU 400 mg/m² IV bolus; continuous-infusion 5-FU 600 mg/m² for 22 hours on days 1 and 2; repeat every 2 weeks; approved first- and second-line therapy
- FOLFOX6—Oxaliplatin, LV, and 5-FU
  - On day 1—Oxaliplatin 85 mg/m² IV over 2 hours; LV 400 mg/m² IV over two hours; 5-FU 400 mg/m² IV bolus
  - On days 1 and 2—5-FU 1,200 mg/m²/day continuous infusion over 48 hours; repeat every 2 weeks
- Cetuximab and irinotecan—Epidermal growth factor receptor–positive disease
  - Cetuximab 400 mg/m² IV first infusion, then 250 mg/m² IV weekly, and irinotecan 350 mg/m² IV every 3 weeks or 125 mg/m² every week for 4 weeks; repeat every 6 weeks
- 5-FU and bevacizumab—First-line therapy
  - Bevacizumab 5 mg/kg IV every 2 weeks, administered with either 5-FU/LV; IFL; FOLFOX; or FOLFIRI

IFL—irinotecan, 5-FU, and LV

Note. Based on information from Kelly & Goldberg, 2005; Meyerhardt & Mayer, 2005; National Comprehensive Cancer Network, 2006b; Viale et al., 2005; Wilkes, 2005; Wilkes & Barton-Burke, 2006.

stage III disease. After resection for stage III colon cancer, administration of 5-FU/LV improves survival (Andre, de Gramont, et al., 2004). In those with advanced CRC, 5-FU prolongs survival by approximately six months (Meyerhardt & Mayer, 2005).

Side effects in patients vary according to the method of administration. Bolus injections daily for five days, repeated every month (the Mayo Clinic regimen), more often lead to neutropenia and stomatitis, whereas weekly doses more often cause diarrhea. Continuous infusions more often lead to palmar-plantar erythrodysesthesia, or hand-foot syndrome (Meyerhardt & Mayer, 2005). Typically, toxicity is lowest with infusional administration of 5-FU (Andre et al., 2003; Sun & Haller, 2005) (see Table 5-1).

Capecitabine

The oral fluoropyrimidine capecitabine (Xeloda®, Hoffmann-LaRoche, Nutley, NJ), a prodrug, converts to 5-FU preferentially in tumor tissue. Its half-life is longer than that of 5-FU, allowing twice-daily administration. In 2001, capecitabine was approved as a first-line treatment for metastatic CRC, achieving response rates superior to those achieved with the Mayo Clinic regimen (26% versus 17%) and demonstrating a nonsignificant trend toward superior three-year survival (Cassidy et al., 2002; Van Cutsem et al., 2001).

One study, the Xeloda in Adjuvant Colon Cancer Therapy (or the X-ACT) trial, randomly assigned 1,987 patients with resected stage III colon cancer to oral capecitabine or IV bolus 5-FU and demonstrated that disease-free survival was

---

Table 5-1. Side Effects of Chemotherapeutic and Biologic Agents Used in Treatment of Colorectal Cancer

Drug	Side Effects
5-fluorouracil (5-FU)	Diarrhea, nausea, vomiting, mucositis, anorexia, pancytopenia, hyperpigmentation with radiation recall, photophobia, integumentary changes including plantar/palmar erythema
Oxaliplatin	Nausea, vomiting, diarrhea, mucositis, pancytopenia, fatigue, anorexia, sensory neuropathy with cold exposure, constipation, increased liver function tests
Cisplatin	Nausea, vomiting, renal and ototoxicity, anorexia, pancytopenia, metallic taste, alopecia, depletion of magnesium, calcium, potassium
Irinotecan	Acute and delayed diarrhea, nausea, vomiting, fatigue, pancytopenia, anorexia, mucositis, skin rash, alopecia
Capecitabine	Pancytopenia, anorexia, mucositis, abdominal pain, fatigue, diarrhea, nausea, vomiting, hand-foot syndrome, integumentary changes
Leucovorin	Mild nausea, vomiting
Floxuridine	Myelosuppression, nausea, vomiting, mucositis or stomatitis of the gastrointestinal tract, alopecia, dermatitis, hepatic dysfunction
Mitomycin-C	Myelosuppression, pulmonary/hepatic/renal toxicity, nausea, vomiting, alopecia, stomatitis
Bevacizumab	Hypertension, fatigue, nausea, vomiting, constipation, anorexia, abdominal pain, leukopenia, asthenia, proteinuria, stomatitis, headache, myalgia, exfoliative dermatitis, gastrointestinal perforation, wound dehiscence
Cetuximab	Acne-like rash, dry skin, fatigue, fever, constipation, abdominal pain

Common protocols
5-FU/leucovorin/oxaliplatin (FOLFOX4)
5-FU/leucovorin
5-FU/leucovorin/irinotecan
5-FU/leucovorin/irinotecan/bevacizumab
Capecitabine
Capecitabine/oxaliplatin
Capecitabine/irinotecan
5-FU/cisplatin
Continuous infusion 5-FU
Hepatic artery infusion—5-FU/leucovorin or floxuridine, continuous 5-FU or floxuridine

Note. From "Colorectal Cancer" (p. 35), by K. Masino in V.J. Kogut and S.L. Luthringer (Eds.), *Nutritional Issues in Cancer Care*, 2005, Pittsburgh, PA: Oncology Nursing Society. Copyright 2005 by the Oncology Nursing Society. Reprinted with permission.

at least equivalent in the two arms. Authors concluded that capecitabine is an effective alternative to IV 5-FU in adjuvant treatment (Twelves et al., 2005).

Side effects of capecitabine included a 17% incidence of grade 3 palmar-plantar erythrodysesthesia, or hand-foot syndrome (Twelves et al., 2005). Most patients required a dose reduction from the 2,500 mg/m^2 to 50%–75% of the full dose, probably necessary because of the amount of folic acid present in the average American diet. Folic acid is an enhancer of 5-FU toxicity (Allegra & Sargent, 2005). For older adults or frail patients, a lower starting dose of 1,000 mg/m^2 twice daily may be better tolerated (Cassidy et al., 2002).

Other studies have shown significant complications of grade 3–4 diarrhea at 1,250 mg/m^2 of capecitabine twice daily when used with oxaliplatin or irinotecan. At doses of 1,000 mg/m^2 twice daily, one phase II trial showed high rates of severe diarrhea requiring hospitalization, which persisted even after dose reduction (Kelly & Goldberg, 2005). Patients require close monitoring for early signs of diarrhea, with dose reductions, hydration, and supportive therapy instituted immediately (see Table 5-1).

Oxaliplatin

Oxaliplatin (Eloxatin®, Sanofi-Aventis, Bridgewater, NJ) is a platinum derivative that induces apoptosis and acts in a synergistic manner with 5-FU/LV. The addition of oxaliplatin to 5-FU and LV doubled the response rate and prolonged progression-free survival among patients with metastatic CRC (de Gramont et al., 2000).

The Multicenter International Study of Oxaliplatin/5-FU/LV in the Adjuvant Treatment of Colon Cancer (MOSAIC) trial, a multinational randomized clinical trial, showed that adding oxaliplatin to infusional 5-FU plus LV (FOLFOX4) significantly prolonged disease-free survival in patients with stage II and III colon cancer and provided a 23% reduction in the risk of recurrence (Andre, Boni, et al., 2004). No significant difference was seen in estimated overall survival at three years between the two groups. In the MOSAIC study, 2,246 patients with surgically resected stage II or III colon cancer were randomly assigned to 5-FU and LV alone (200 mg/m^2 LV IV and bolus of 400 mg 5-FU/m^2, followed by a 22-hour infusion of 600 mg/m^2 of 5-FU given on two consecutive days every 14 days for 12 cycles) or with oxaliplatin (same 5-FU/LV regimen and a two-hour infusion of 85 mg/m^2 oxaliplatin day 1 given simultaneously with LV). The safety of infused 5-FU, LV, and oxaliplatin was acceptable, but peripheral neuropathy, myelosuppression, and GI distress were more common in the oxaliplatin arm. Neutropenia, diarrhea, and vomiting were the most frequent grade 3 or 4 toxicities in the group receiving oxaliplatin (see Table 5-1). Of the 12.4% of patients who had a grade 3 peripheral neuropathy during treatment, grade 3 symptoms still were present in eight patients at six months post-treatment. It should be noted that 92% of patients had some degree of neuropathy on the oxaliplatin arm. Results are impressive, and this trial resulted in approval

by the U.S. Food and Drug Administration of oxaliplatin for adjuvant treatment with 5-FU/LV, and this combination became a new standard adjuvant therapy for patients with stage III colon cancers (Andre, Boni, et al.). Overall survival differences will be released soon. The addition of oxaliplatin to weekly bolus fluorouracil and leucovorin significantly improved three-year disease-free survival for patients with stage II and III colon cancer (Wolmark, 2005).

The FOLFOX4 regimen, bolus 5-FU/LV, infusional 5-FU, and oxaliplatin, has resulted in superior response rates in advanced CRC than 5-FU/LV alone. These results have been noted when the regimen is given as first- or second-line therapy. In patients with stage III disease, FOLFOX4 resulted in four-year recurrence-free survival in 70% of cases, compared to 61% in the 5-FU/LV arm (Andre, Boni, et al., 2004). For stage II patients, disease-free survival was 81%, versus 85% in the FOLFOX4 arm (Andre, Boni, et al.). Because of these data, FOLFOX4 is the recommended treatment for early-stage colon cancer (NCCN, 2006b). In the metastatic setting, patients who received FOLFOX have demonstrated a greater increase in median survival than regimens containing irinotecan (Kelly & Goldberg, 2005). FOLFOX4 has become standard first-line therapy in the metastatic setting, and oxaliplatin is approved for adjuvant therapy as well.

Oxaliplatin induces frequent, transient paresthesias during or shortly after the first minutes of infusion. Noted in the hands, feet, and perioral regions, the paresthesias are exacerbated by exposure to cold, called cold-induced dysthesia. Simply holding a cold can of soda can exacerbate the symptom. The neurotoxicity can increase in intensity as treatment continues and can interfere with activities of daily living. Some patients describe a feeling of being unable to catch their breath without having any supporting physical manifestations. This is known as acute pharyngolaryngeal dysthesia and occurs in 1%–2% of patients (Thomas, Quinn, Schuler, & Grem, 2003). After prolonged therapy (800 mg/m^2), patients may have a sensory neuropathy that continues after the treatment is infused. This neuropathy abates after cessation of therapy (de Gramont et al., 2000). Injury prevention will be necessary if the patient develops sensory neuropathy. Patients should take caution against burning hands while cooking; full prevention techniques with use of topical or adjuvant analgesics may be indicated (Almadrones & Arcot, 1999). Reports have emerged about calcium and magnesium infusions and oral calcium to modulate this side effect, but these are anecdotal (Gamelin et al., 2004; Saif, 2004). Oxaliplatin increases the incidence of neutropenia and diarrhea over 5-FU/LV alone (Kelly & Goldberg, 2005).

Irinotecan

Irinotecan (Camptosar®, Pfizer Oncology, New York, NY), a topoisomerase I inhibitor, causes DNA fragmentation and cell death and was approved for the treatment of metastatic CRC in 1997. Subsequently, the addition of irinotecan to 5-FU/LV was shown to increase survival duration when used as first-line treatment in metastatic CRC (Douillard et al., 2000; Saltz et al., 2000) (see Figure 5-7). However, Saltz et al. (2004) reported results of another trial that randomly assigned patients (N = 1,264) with stage III colon cancer to receive irinotecan and bolus 5-FU/LV or bolus 5-FU/LV alone for six months. Results of this study demonstrated that patients in the irinotecan arm had increased rates of febrile neutropenia and treatment-related death and at three years showed no difference in overall survival over the 5-FU/LV–alone arm. The authors concluded that IFL should not have been an option for adjuvant treatment. FOLFIRI (irinotecan, LV, and 5-FU), with or without bevacizumab, may be a treatment of choice as neoadjuvant therapy in patients with resectable metastatic disease to the liver (NCCN, 2006b). FOLFIRI also is a treatment option as primary therapy in advanced disease if patients can withstand intense treatment (NCCN, 2006b).

Side effects of irinotecan include diarrhea, with early and late onset, bone marrow suppression, GI distress in the form of nausea and vomiting, and alopecia. Acute onset diarrhea usually is transient and is accompanied by cholinergic symptoms such as flushing, salivating, and hyperperistalsis (see Table 5-1). Atropine can be used to treat or prevent the acute form (Wilkes, 2005). The delayed diarrhea requires patient education and close monitoring. The patient can manage uncomplicated cases at home with intensive loperamide, but he or she should contact the healthcare provider if diarrhea persists. Adding irinotecan to 5-FU/LV increases the severity of diarrhea and myelosuppression and has been documented to increase patient mortality in one trial (Kelly & Goldberg, 2005). Bolus dosing of 5-FU seems to have contributed to this effect because of its higher incidence of neutropenia.

For patients who have demonstrated severe toxicity after irinotecan treatment, particularly severe neutropenia, the patient may have a genetic mutation known as UGT1A1 polymorphism. This syndrome is associated with hyperbilirubinemia, and patients who have this polymorphism or who have Gilbert disease, another hyperbilirubinemia syndrome, should not receive irinotecan (Desai, Innocenti, & Ratain, 2003; Innocenti et al., 2004; NCCN, 2006b).

Cetuximab

Cetuximab (Erbitux®, ImClone/Bristol-Myers Squibb, Princeton, NJ) is a monoclonal antibody against epidermal growth factor receptors (EGFRs). It has shown activity for patients who have irinotecan-refractory metastatic CRC and is approved for use in the metastatic setting. In a large clinical trial, patients refractory to irinotecan received either cetuximab with irinotecan or cetuximab alone. The group receiving the cetuximab with irinotecan had double the tumor regression (radiographically) compared to those who received cetuximab alone (Cunningham et al., 2004). Patients in these trials have been limited to those with EGFR expression, but that may not be a factor in determining response. Recent data confirm that the presence of EGFR mutation does not determine response to cetuximab (Chung et al., 2005).

A study comparing cetuximab, bevacizumab, and irinotecan to cetuximab and bevacizumab appeared to show that bevacizumab added to the efficacy of cetuximab, and cetuximab/irinotecan, in irinotecan-refractory, bevacizumab-naïve patients. Toxicities included rash, neutropenia, and diarrhea, all of which were more significant in the patients receiving all three drugs (Saltz et al., 2005).

Side effects consist of an acne-like rash, which can be severe (Viale, Fung, & Zitella, 2005), and drying of the skin (see Table 5-1). Eighty percent of patients develop some type of rash. The development and severity of the rash may be correlated with the likelihood of having an objective response (Meyerhardt & Mayer, 2005). Hypersensitivity reactions also can occur in 20% of patients and can be treated with a premedication of diphenhydramine. Hypomagnesemia also has been reported (Schrag, Chung, Flombaum, & Saltz, 2005).

Bevacizumab

Angiogenesis, the process of new blood vessel growth, is critical for the growth of tumors, and recent success in blocking tumor-related angiogenesis is promising. Bevacizumab (Avastin®, Genentech, South San Francisco, CA) is a monoclonal antibody against vascular endothelial growth factor (VEGF). The VEGF family consists of six proteins, including VEGF A, B, C, D, E, and placental growth factor. VEGF A is the protein commonly referred to as VEGF and is a key factor in controlling blood vessel growth (Collins & Hurwitz, 2005); it is overexpressed in many tumors. Bevacizumab has been studied in several trials of patients having initial therapy for metastatic disease and is found to increase response rate and prolong overall survival when added to IFL (Hurwitz et al., 2004) and to improve response rates when added to 5-FU/LV alone (Kabbinavar et al., 2003) (see Figure 5-7). In a study by Hurwitz et al., response rates were 44.8% in the bevacizumab arm compared to 34.8% in the IFL arm (p = 0.004). It has been approved for use with any 5-FU regimen in patients with advanced CRC. Bevacizumab is not active as a single agent, nor is it effective if reused after initial treatment (Saltz et al., 2005). Adding bevacizumab to FOLFOX or capecitabine/oxaliplatin combinations also improved response rates (Hochster et al., 2005). Other agents are being evaluated in CRC for antiangiogenesis activity. Vatalanib inhibits VEGF by inhibiting angiogenesis, and thalidomide also is being evaluated for its well-known antiangiogenesis properties (Collins & Hurwitz).

Side effects of bevacizumab include nosebleeds, hypertension, and wound dehiscence, with epistaxis lasting < 5 minutes without intervention being the most common (Hurwitz et al., 2004) (see Table 5-1). The hypertension is usually reversible, responsive to antihypertensive medications, and may be accompanied by proteinuria (Hurwitz et al.; Wilkes, 2005). Bevacizumab has a significant side effect of risk for GI perforation. This occurred in six patients (with one fatality) receiving bevacizumab in the IFL/bevacizumab study (Hurwitz et al.). Although this may be related to the biology of wound healing, it is unclear what period of time is optimum between surgery and receipt of bevacizumab. Hemorrhage and arterial clots also have been reported.

Summary

To summarize, an extraordinary amount of data recently have emerged on treatment of colon cancer. New agents, new surgical techniques, and various permutations of both have provided healthcare professionals with a variety of treatment options. Consideration of the patient's physical condition, tumor characteristics, and lifestyle needs will be paramount in the treatment options selected.

For patients with high-risk T3 or T4 tumors (N0M0 or T 1-4, N1-2, M0), treatment may involve 5-FU/LV, FOLFOX, or capecitabine. Selection of which version of FOLFOX is used often is dependent on local preferences.

For patients with resectable liver or lung metastases, treatment may involve 5-FU/LV, FOLFOX, or capecitabine, hepatic artery infusion therapy with or without 5-FU/LV, or infusional 5-FU. FUDR (fluorodeoxyuridine) via hepatic artery infusion plus systemic chemotherapy is superior to systemic chemotherapy alone after hepatic resection. Neoadjuvant chemotherapy with FOLFOX or FOLFIRI with or without bevacizumab may make resection possible.

For patients with metastatic disease, FOLFOX and bevacizumab, FOLFIRI and bevacizumab, IFL and bevacizumab, or 5-FU/LV with or without bevacizumab may be preferred.

Patients receiving combination regimens and having received all three drugs (5-FU, oxaliplatin, irinotecan) exhibit improved response rates and survival (Grothey & Sargent, 2005; NCCN, 2006b).

Rectal Cancer

As previously described, patients with tumors that are larger than T2 will be treated with radiation therapy plus chemotherapy. NCCN guidelines (2006c) currently recommend the following treatment.

- For patients with T1-2, N0, or M0 tumors, local excision or transabdominal resection is recommended.
- For patients with resectable T3 tumors with negative nodes or any size tumor with positive nodes: preoperative radiotherapy with concurrent chemotherapy (continuous-infusion 5-FU) or transabdominal resection, followed by postoperative adjuvant chemotherapy of 5-FU, with or without LV, or FOLFOX or capecitabine. Preoperative radiation therapy with concomitant continuous-infusion 5-FU is useful in increasing the resectability of adenocarcinoma of the rectum and may be more effective than postoperative radiation in reducing local recurrence (Arnoletti & Bland, 2006; NCCN, 2006c).
- For patients with advanced disease, recommendations include resection of the primary lesion and any metastases

or continuous-infusion 5-FU/pelvic radiation, bolus 5-FU/LV with radiation, or FOLFOX, FOLFIRI, or IFL with or without bevacizumab (NCCN, 2006c).

- Radiation side effects to the rectal area include skin alterations, diarrhea, and adhesions. Preoperative radiation has been reported to have lower rates of side effects and improved sphincter preservation rates (Minsky et al., 1992).

Radiation therapy, particularly to the perineal and perianal areas, can be accompanied by significant side effects. Abdominal cramping, diarrhea, tenesmus, pruritus, and desquamation are possible. Teaching the patient appropriate skin care is imperative in preventing complications. Cleansing with tepid water and mild soap, using cotton undergarments, and avoiding heavy, perfumed lotions will promote comfort. Moist desquamation can be accompanied by weeping and abscess formation; sitz baths may be helpful. Fatigue and persistent diarrhea can be debilitating. A low-residue diet, adequate hydration, and frequent rest periods should be encouraged.

With the increasing use of combined chemotherapy/radiation therapies, the incidence of radiation enteritis has increased. Acute radiation enteritis may appear at any time after the first fraction (radiation dose given in one day) but is more commonly seen during the third week, with an incidence of 20%–70% (Nguyen & Antoine, 2002). Malabsorptive diarrhea from loss of intestinal crypt cells, cramping, diarrhea, nausea, and decreased absorption of B vitamins commonly is seen but usually subsides after the radiation is completed. Chronic radiation enteritis develops in a small number of patients (1%–15%) who are predisposed by age, vascular disease, or postoperative radiation (Nguyen & Antoine). Clinical signs and symptoms are diagnostic, but mucosal ulceration and thickening of intestinal loops also may be seen radiologically with chronic enteritis. Acute enteritis usually resolves with supportive care, but some patients may require parenteral fluid replacement.

Regional Liver Therapy

More than 50% of patients with CRC develop liver metastases (Leonard, Brenner, & Kemeny, 2005). Regional therapy to the liver for treatment of metastases is an increasingly important modality in advanced CRC. Surgical resection of metastases is the best chance for cure, but only 10%–20% of patients with colorectal liver metastases are eligible for such resections (Adam et al., 2004). For patients with nonresectable metastases, other options are available.

Hepatic arterial infusion (HAI) chemotherapy delivers chemotherapy, usually floxuridine FUDR, directly to the hepatic artery. Studies have shown a survival advantage in patients who received HAI over chemotherapy with 5-FU/LV alone (Leonard et al., 2004) and improved resectability of metastases after HAI and systemic chemotherapy with oxaliplatin-based systemic therapy (Leonard et al., 2004).

Complications of HAI include catheter displacement, hepatic artery occlusion, thrombosis, and bleeding (Leonard,

Brenner, & Kemeny, 2005). Other side effects include nausea and vomiting, chemical hepatitis, and bone marrow toxicity (Leonard et al., 2005). Pain control is essential, and the nurse should assess for pain frequently. Oral and parenteral therapies for pain may be indicated (Cahill, 2005).

Radiofrequency ablation is an effective local therapy that causes intense intratumoral heat, under MRI or CT guidance, using a specially designed probe (see Figure 5-8). Intraoperative ultrasonography also may be used to guide the needle into the tumor, where electrical current is delivered, causing frictional heat and a zone of ischemia within the tumor. Grounding pads are placed on the patient to complete an electrical circuit and prevent patient burns (Locklin & Wood, 2005).

Patients may experience diaphoreses from increased body temperatures during the procedure. If not done under general anesthesia, pain control may be required to facilitate patient comfort and compliance with the procedure. The grounding pads should be assessed regularly during the procedure to ensure that the patient's skin is not hot or inflamed. Postoperatively, the patient should be placed on his or her right side for at least an hour and should be observed for bleeding, changes in vital signs, or peritoneal hemorrhage. Postoperative hydration to flush byproducts of ablation and observation for postablation syndrome, which is similar to tumor lysis syndrome, should be performed. Symptoms of postablation syndrome may include low-grade fever, aches, flu-like symptoms, and malaise (Locklin & Wood, 2005; Melliza & Woodall, 2000). Other options include cryosurgery and ethanol injections.

Anal Cancers

Small, localized anal cancers may be fully treated with surgical excision. Chemotherapy given concurrently with radiation is the preferred therapy for most patients with anal cancer. A large randomized trial demonstrated that the use of mitomycin with irradiation and 5-FU was more successful than radiation and 5-FU alone in improving colostomy-free survival (Ellerhorn, Cullinane, Coia, & Alberts, 2004). Cisplatin and 5-FU combinations also have shown effectiveness (NCCN, 2006a).

Gastrointestinal Stromal Tumors

Introduction

Gastrointestinal stromal tumors (GIST) are soft-tissue sarcomas occurring in the GI tract and are uncommon, accounting for 0.2% of all GI malignancies. However, they are the most common sarcoma of the abdomen (Raut et al., 2006). Recent progress in diagnosis of these tumors has led to an increase in the estimated incidence of 5,000 new cases per year in the United States (Demetri, 2005). GIST occurs predominantly in adults from age 50–80, with a peak age in the 60s, and occurs more often in men (Corless, Fletcher, & Heinrich, 2004; Demetri).

Characteristics

The majority of GISTs develop in the stomach (40%–70%), followed by 20%–40% in the small intestine, 5%–15% in the colon and rectum, and < 5% in the esophagus (Raut et al., 2006; Savage & Antman, 2002). GISTs also can occur in the mesentery or retroperitoneum (Demetri, 2005). Tumors can take a variable course, with some remaining stable for years and others rapidly progressing to metastatic disease. Some data suggest that GISTs originate from CD34+ stem cells

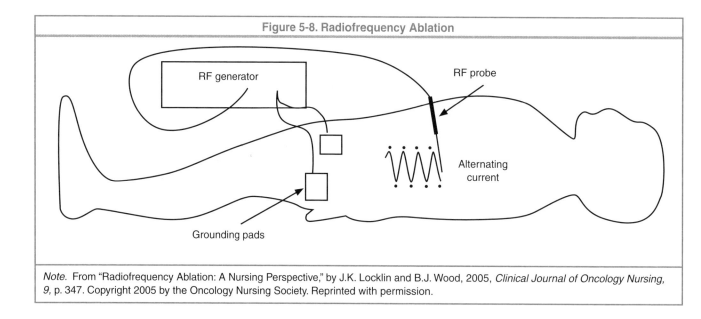

Figure 5-8. Radiofrequency Ablation

RF generator

RF probe

Alternating current

Grounding pads

Note. From "Radiofrequency Ablation: A Nursing Perspective," by J.K. Locklin and B.J. Wood, 2005, *Clinical Journal of Oncology Nursing, 9,* p. 347. Copyright 2005 by the Oncology Nursing Society. Reprinted with permission.

in the gut wall, which then differentiate into interstitial cells of Cajal (ICCs). ICCs are pacemaker cells in the gut that are active in peristalsis by linking active smooth muscle with the autonomic nervous system. There are biologic similarities between ICCs and GIST cells. Both cells express KIT, a transmembrane tyrosine kinase receptor (Demetri). KIT (CD 117) is expressed by mast cells, some stem cells, and ICCs. Mutations in KIT, a proto-oncogene that affects the tyrosine kinase receptor, are found in 90%–95% of GISTs (Demetri). It had been thought that tumors with the mutation were more often high-grade with more frequent recurrences than those tumors without the mutation, but subsequent research has shown that even the smallest GISTs have KIT mutations (Demetri). All GISTs have some degree of malignant potential and are classified as low, intermediate, or high risk (Griffin, St. Amand, & Demetri, 2005).

Diagnosis and Staging

Clinical presentation can vary from asymptomatic to acutely symptomatic if tumors are a large size or obstructive. Patients may describe pain, nausea, vomiting, weight loss, and anorexia. The majority of metastases are intra-abdominal to the liver or peritoneal cavity and rarely by lymphatic spread.

Diagnostic tests include CT scan to evaluate the primary tumor and magnetic resonance imaging to detect hepatic metastases. Biopsy and expert pathologic review are essential for diagnosis. Immunohistochemical assays usually demonstrate CD 117 antigen expression, a marker for the presence of the KIT protein, which the majority (85%) of GISTs expresses (Demetri, 2005; Raut et al., 2006). KIT expression occurs infrequently in most other tumor types, and with the exception of GISTs, KIT gene mutations are rare (Went et al., 2004). Positron-emission tomography with F-fluorodeoxyglucose can provide useful information on the extent of disease and metabolic activity of the tumor (Demetri).

Prognostic Factors

Survival rates are associated with location; esophageal and stomach tumors have the highest survival rates, whereas small intestine tumors have the lowest (Savage & Antman, 2002). The most reliable prognostic factors are size of the tumor and the mitotic index, which is the proliferative activity of the tumor (Demetri, 2005). Prior to targeted therapies, survival from GIST was poor, with a life expectancy of two years for patients with unresectable disease (Demetri; Raut et al., 2006).

Surgical Management

Small, localized tumors can be surgically resected. Surgery has not been a preferred treatment for patients with metastatic disease because of multifocal liver and peritoneal metastases. Disease initially judged as unresectable may become amenable to surgical resection after treatment with imatinib, and debulking procedures in patients on kinase inhibitor therapies are associated with prolonged overall survival (Raut et al., 2006).

Chemotherapeutic Management

Up until 2002, treatment of advanced disease (metastatic or unresectable) with standard chemotherapeutic agents was poor, and resistance to chemotherapy occurred rapidly. Imatinib mesylate (Gleevec®, Novartis Pharmaceuticals Corp., East Hanover, NJ) is a drug that inhibits the tyrosine kinase activity of KIT. It had been successfully used in treatment of chronic myeloid leukemia. Studies on a leukemia cell line with a KIT mutation similar to that of GIST showed that imatinib mesylate successfully inhibited KIT proteins. Research expanded into clinical trials on the use of this agent in patients with GISTs. Multiple trials demonstrated substantial activity of imatinib in metastatic GIST, producing objective responses and symptom control, with median time to objective response being more than three months (Demetri, 2005; Demetri et al., 2002). On the basis of these data, the U.S. Food and Drug Administration approved imatinib for treatment of metastatic or unresectable GIST in 2002. Adverse effects of treatment are mild: edema (74%, especially in the periorbital area), diarrhea (45%), myalgia (40%), skin rash (30%), and headache (25%) (Demetri). However, 5% of patients developed hemorrhage from abdominal or GI sites (Demetri). Most experts believe that treatment with imatinib should be lifelong in order to maintain control of GIST. Resistance to imatinib can occur and is evidenced by rapid progression of disease. Acquired resistance to imatinib is expected to increase (Demetri).

In a phase III trial (N = 312), the multitargeted therapy, sunitinib (Sutent®, Pfizer Inc., New York, NY), demonstrated efficacy in patients with imatinib-resistant GIST. This drug inhibits several kinases that play a role in promoting cancer growth and angiogenesis. Significant improvements in survival (50% lower relative risk of death) and progression-free survival (6.3 versus 1.5 months) were seen in patients receiving sunitinib compared to those given a placebo (Demetri, van Oosterom, & Blackstein, 2005). Sunitinib was approved for treatment of metastatic or unresectable GISTs in January 2006 (Raut et al., 2006). Adverse effects were usually mild, and included fatigue, hypertension, diarrhea, skin discoloration, mouth irritation, weakness, and altered taste.

Nursing Considerations

The dosage of imatinib is 400 mg or 600 mg po daily, administered continuously as long as the disease is stable or responding to therapy (Demetri, 2005). Some trials have shown a modest benefit in favor of the larger dose in terms of survival, but they showed a higher incidence of adverse effects as well. These therapies are long-term, and educating patients about the importance of compliance is essential. Pills come in 400 mg oblong tablets or 100 mg round tablets, and nurses and patients should be aware of this difference (Griffin et al., 2005). CYP3A4 is the major enzyme responsible for metabolism of imatinib, and inhibitors or inducers of CYP isoenzymes can lead to drug interactions. Drugs that may increase imatinib plasma concentrations include ketoconazole, itraconazole, erythromycin, and clarithromycin. Drugs that decrease imatinib plasma concentrations include dexamethasone, phenytoin, rifampicin, phenobarbital, or St. John's wort. Imatinib increases the plasma levels of simvastatin by two- to threefold, and warfarin should not be administered to patients taking imatinib (Griffin et al.; Novartis Pharmaceuticals Corp., 2005). The dosage for sunitinib is 50 mg once daily on a schedule of four weeks on treatment followed by two weeks off. An increase or decrease in dose is recommended in 12.5 mg increments based on the patient's tolerance. CYP precautions also are recommended for sunitinib (U.S. Food and Drug Administration, 2006b).

Teaching patients to restrict salt in the diet is helpful in controlling edema, and patients should weigh themselves regularly and report any significant weight changes. Diuretics may be advisable if patients have fluid retention. Skin reactions such as rash, pruritis, dryness, or lightening of skin tone have occurred in people with darker complexions. Moisturizing the skin and using antihistamines are effective measures. Nausea, vomiting, GI distress, and diarrhea can occur. The drug should be taken with food and eight ounces of water. Grapefruit juice should be avoided because it inhibits CYP3A4 and could alter blood levels of imatinib. Antiemetics or loperamide may be used as needed. Patients who are nursing or pregnant should not take imatinib (Griffin et al., 2005).

Blood pressure monitoring is recommended during treatment with sunitinib, and high blood pressure can be treated with standard therapies. Both imatinib and sunitinib have been associated with cardiac abnormalities. Imatinib has been associated with cardiotoxicity from tyrosine kinase inhibition (Kerkelä et al., 2006) and can lead to left ventricular dysfunction and congestive heart failure. Sunitinib has been associated with left ventricular dysfunction in patients with cardiac histories. Baseline evaluation of ejection fraction should be considered in patients without cardiac risk factors. Treatment should be discontinued if congestive heart failure develops, and the dose should be reduced in patients who have ejection fractions between 20%–50% below baseline (U.S. Food and Drug Administration, 2000a). Incidence of this effect is very low.

Summary

Significant advances in treatment of colon, rectal, and anal cancers have been described. Data continue to rapidly emerge, and randomized clinical trials will demonstrate ultimate efficacy in terms of patient survival, response rates, and quality of life.

References

Adam, R., Pascal, G., Castaing, D., Azoulay, D., Delvart, V., Paule, B., et al. (2004). Tumor progression while on chemotherapy. *Annals of Surgery, 240,* 1052–1061.

Alberts, S.R., Donohue, J.H., Mahoney, M.R., Horvath, W.L., Sternfeld, W.C., Dakhil, S.R., et al. (2003). Liver resection after 5-fluorouracil, leucovorin and oxaliplatin for patients with metastatic colorectal cancer (MCRC) limited to the liver: A North Central Cancer Treatment Group (NCCTG) phase II study [Abstract 1053]. *Proceedings of the American Society of Clinical Oncology, 22,* 263.

Allegra, C., & Sargent, D.J. (2005). Adjuvant therapy for colon cancer—The pace quickens. *New England Journal of Medicine, 352,* 2746–2748.

Almadrones, L., & Arcot, R. (1999). Patient guide to peripheral neuropathy. *Oncology Nursing Forum, 26,* 1359–1361.

Andre, T., Boni, C., Mounedji-Boudiaf, L., Navarro, M., Tabernero, J., Hickish, T., et al. (2004). Oxaliplatin, fluorouracil, and leucovorin as adjuvant treatment for colon cancer. *New England Journal of Medicine, 350,* 2343–2351.

Andre, T., Colin, P., Louvet, C., Gamelin, E., Bouche, O., Achille, E., et al. (2003). Semi-monthly versus monthly regimen of fluorouracil and leucovorin administered for 24 or 36 weeks as adjuvant therapy in stage II and III colon cancer: Results of a randomized trial. *Journal of Clinical Oncology, 21,* 2896–2903.

Andre, T., de Gramont, A., Study Group of Clinical Research in Radiotherapies Oncology, & Oncology Multidisciplinary Research Group. (2004). An overview of adjuvant systemic chemotherapy for colon cancer. *Clinical Colorectal Cancer, 4*(Suppl. 1), S22–S28.

Arnoletti, J., & Bland, K. (2006). Neoadjuvant and adjuvant therapy for rectal cancer. *Surgical Oncology Clinics of North America, 15,* 147–157.

Benson, A.B., Schrag, D., Somerfield, M.R., Cohen, A.M., Figueredo, A.T., Flynn, P.J., et al. (2004). ASCO recommendations on adjuvant chemotherapy for stage II colon cancer. *Journal of Clinical Oncology, 22,* 3408–3419.

Bilchik, A.J., Poston, G., Curley, S.A., Strasberg, S., Saltz, L., Adam, R., et al. (2005). Neoadjuvant chemotherapy for metastatic colon cancer: A cautionary note. *Journal of Clinical Oncology, 23,* 9073–9078.

Cahill, B. (2005). Management of patients who have undergone hepatic artery chemoembolization. *Clinical Journal of Oncology Nursing, 9,* 69–75.

Cassidy, J., Twelves, C., Van Cutsem, E., Hoff, P., Bajetta, E., Boyer, M., et al. (2002). First-line oral capecitabine therapy in metastatic colorectal cancer: A favorable safety profile compared with intravenous 5-fluorouracil/leucovorin. *Annals of Oncology, 13,* 566–575.

Chung, K., Shia, J., Kemeny, N., Shah, M., Schwartz, G., Tse, A., et al. (2005). Cetuximab shows activity in colorectal cancer patients with tumors that do not express the epidermal growth factor receptor by immunohistochemistry. *Journal of Clinical Oncology, 23,* 1803–1810.

Clinical Outcomes of Surgical Therapy Study Group. (2004). A comparison of laparoscopically assisted and open colectomy for colon cancer. *New England Journal of Medicine, 350,* 2050–2059.

Collins, T.S., & Hurwitz, H.I. (2005). Targeting vascular endothelial growth factor and angiogenesis for the treatment of colorectal cancer. *Seminars in Oncology, 32,* 61–68.

Corless, C., Fletcher, J., & Heinrich, M. (2004). Biology of gastrointestinal stromal tumors. *Journal of Clinical Oncology, 22,* 3813–3825.

Cunningham, D., Humblet, Y., Siena, S., Khayat, D., Bleiberg, H., Santoro, A., et al. (2004). Cetuximab monotherapy and cetuximab plus irinotecan in irinotecan-refractory metastatic colorectal cancer. *New England Journal of Medicine, 351,* 337–345.

de Gramont, A., Figer, A., Seymour, M., Homerin, M., Hmissi, A., Cassidy, J., et al. (2000). Leucovorin and fluorouracil with or without oxaliplatin as first-line treatment in advanced colorectal cancer. *Journal of Clinical Oncology, 18,* 2938–2947.

Demetri, G. (2005). Gastrointestinal stromal tumors. In V.T. DeVita, S. Hellman, & S. Rosenberg (Eds.), *Cancer: Principles and practice of oncology* (7th ed., pp. 1050–1060). Philadelphia: Lippincott Williams & Wilkins.

Demetri, G., von Mehren, M., Blanke, C., Van Den Abbeele, A., Eisenberg, B., Roberts, P., et al. (2002). Efficacy and safety of imatinib mesylate in advanced gastrointestinal stromal tumors. *New England Journal of Medicine, 347,* 472–480.

Demetri, G., van Oosterom, A., & Blackstein, M. (2005). Phase 3, multicenter, randomized, double-blind, placebo-controlled trial of SU11248 in patients following failure of imatinib for metastatic GIST [Abstract]. *Journal of Clinical Oncology, 23,* 308S.

Desai, A., Innocenti, F., & Ratain, M. (2003). Pharmacogenomics: Road to anticancer therapeutics nirvana? *Oncogene, 22,* 6621–6628.

Douillard, J., Cunningham, D., Roth, A., Navarro, M., James, R., Karasek, P., et al. (2000). Irinotecan combined with fluorouracil compared with fluorouracil alone as first-line treatment for metastatic colorectal cancer: A multicentre randomized trial. *Lancet, 355,* 1041–1047.

Ellerhorn, J., Cullinane, C., Coia, L., & Alberts, S. (2004). Colorectal and anal cancers. In R. Pazdur, L. Coia, W. Hoskins, & L. Wagman (Eds.), *Cancer management: A multidisciplinary approach* (8th ed., pp. 323–355). Melville, NY: F.A. Davis.

Gamelin, L., Boisdron-Celle, M., Delva, R., Guerin-Meyer, V., Ifrah, N., Morel, A., et al. (2004). Prevention of oxaliplatin-related neurotoxicity by calcium and magnesium infusions. *Clinical Cancer Research, 10,* 4055–4061.

Gray, R.G., Barnwell, J., Hills, R., McConkey, C., Williams, N., Kerr, D., et al. (2004). QUASAR: A randomized study of adjuvant chemotherapy (CT) vs observation including 3238 colorectal cancer patients [Abstract 3501]. *Journal of Clinical Oncology, 22*(Suppl. 14), 3501.

Greene, F.L., Page, D.L., Fleming, I.D., & Fritz, A. (2002). *AJCC cancer staging manual* (6th ed.). New York: Springer-Verlag.

Greene, F.L., Stewart, A., & Norton, H. (2002). A new TNM staging strategy for node-positive (stage III) colon cancer: An analysis of 50,042 patients. *Annals of Surgery, 236,* 416–421.

Griffin, J., St. Amand, M., & Demetri, G. (2005). Nursing implications of imatinib as molecularly targeted therapy for gastrointestinal stromal tumors. *Clinical Journal of Oncology Nursing, 9,* 161–169.

Grothey, A., & Sargent, D. (2005). Overall survival of patients with advanced colorectal cancer correlates with availability of fluorouracil, irinotecan and oxaliplatin regardless of whether doublet or single agent therapy is used first line. *Journal of Clinical Oncology, 23,* 9441–9442.

Haller, D., Catalano, P., MacDonald, S., O'Rourke, M., Frontiera, M., Jackson, D., et al. (1998). Phase III study of fluorouracil, leucovorin, and levamisole in high-risk stage II and III colon cancer: Final report of Intergroup 0089 [Abstract No. 982]. *Proceedings of the American Society of Clinical Oncology, 17,* 265a.

Hochster, H.S., Welles, L., Hart, L., Ramanathan, R.K., Hainsworth, J., Jirau-Lucca, G., et al. (2005). Safety and efficacy of bevacizumab when added to oxaliplatin/fluoropyrimidine regimens as first-line treatment of metastatic colorectal cancer: TREE 1 & 2 Studies. *Journal of Clinical Oncology, 23*(Suppl. 16S), 3515.

Hurwitz, H., Fehrenbacher, L., Novotny, W., Cartwright, T., Hainsworth, J., Heim, W., et al. (2004). Bevacizumab plus irinotecan, fluorouracil, and leucovorin for metastatic colorectal cancer. *New England Journal of Medicine, 350,* 2335–2342.

Innocenti, F., Undevia, S.D., Iyer, L., Chen, P.X., Das, S., Kocherginsky, M., et al. (2004). Genetic variants in the UDP-glucuronosyltransferase 1A1 gene predict the risk of severe neutropenia of irinotecan. *Journal of Clinical Oncology, 22,* 1382–1388.

Kabbinavar, F., Hurwitz, H., Fehrenbacher, L., Meropol, N.J., Novotny, W.F., Lieberman, G., et al. (2003). Phase II randomized trial comparing bevacizumab plus fluorouracil with FU/LV alone in patients with metastatic colorectal cancer. *Journal of Clinical Oncology, 21,* 60–65.

Kapiteijn, E., Marijnen, C., Nagtegaal, I., Putter, H., Steup, W., Wiggers, T., et al. (2001). Preoperative radiotherapy combined with total mesorectal excision for resectable rectal cancer. *New England Journal of Medicine, 345,* 638–646.

Kelly, H., & Goldberg, R. (2005). Systemic therapy for metastatic colorectal cancer: Current options, current evidence. *Journal of Clinical Oncology, 23,* 4553–4560.

Kerkelä, R., Grazette, L., Yacobi, R., Iliescu, C., Patten, R., Beahm, C., et al. (2006). Cardiotoxicity of the cancer therapeutic agent imatinib mesylate. *Nature Medicine, 12,* 908–916.

Laurie, J.A., Moertel, C.G., Fleming, T.R., Wieand, H.S., Leigh, J.E., Rubin, J., et al. (1989). Surgical adjuvant therapy of large-bowel carcinoma: An evaluation of levamisole and the combination of levamisole and fluorouracil. The North Central Cancer Treatment Group and the Mayo Clinic. *Annals of Oncology, 7,* 1447–1456.

Leonard, G., Brenner, B., & Kemeny, N. (2005). Neoadjuvant chemotherapy before liver resection for patients with unresectable liver metastases from colorectal carcinoma. *Journal of Clinical Oncology, 23,* 2038–2048.

Leonard, G., Fong, Y., Jarnagin, W., Harris, R., Schwartz, L., D'Angelica, M., et al. (2004). Liver resection after hepatic arterial infusion plus systemic oxaliplatin combinations in pretreated patients with extensive unresectable colorectal liver metastases [Abstract 3542]. *Proceedings of the American Society of Clinical Oncology, 23,* 256.

Le Voyer, T.E., Sigurdson, E.R., Hanlon, A.L., Mayer, R.J., Macdonald, J.S., Catalano, P.J., et al. (2003). Colon cancer survival is associated with increasing number of lymph nodes analyzed: A secondary survey of intergroup trial INT-0089. *Journal of Clinical Oncology, 21,* 2912–2919.

Libutti, S., Saltz, L., Rustgi, A., & Tepper, J. (2005). Cancer of the colon. In V.T. DeVita, S. Hellman, & S.A. Rosenberg (Eds.), *Cancer: Principles and practice of oncology* (7th ed., pp. 1061–1109). Philadelphia: Lippincott Williams & Wilkins.

Libutti, S., Tepper, J., Saltz, L., & Rustgi, A. (2005). Cancer of the rectum. In V.T. DeVita, S. Hellman, & S. Rosenberg (Eds.), *Cancer: Principles and practice of oncology* (7th ed., pp. 1110–1124). Philadelphia: Lippincott Williams & Wilkins.

Locklin, J., & Wood, B. (2005). Radiofrequency ablation: A nursing perspective. *Clinical Journal of Oncology Nursing, 23,* 210–214.

Manning, M. (2004). Management of patients with intestinal and rectal disorders. In S. Smeltzer & B. Bare (Eds.), *Brunner and Suddarth's textbook of medical surgical nursing* (10th ed., pp. 1028–1071). Philadelphia: Lippincott Williams & Wilkins.

Melliza, D., & Woodall, M. (2000). Radiofrequency ablation of liver tumors: The complementary roles of the clinic and research nurse. *Gastroenterology Nursing, 23,* 210–214.

Meyerhardt, J.A., & Mayer, R.J. (2005). Systemic therapy for colorectal cancer. *New England Journal of Medicine, 352,* 476–487.

Minsky, B., Cohen, A., Kemeny, N., Enker, W.E., Kelsen, D.P., Reichman, B., et al. (1992). Combined modality therapy of rectal cancer: Decreased acute toxicity with the pre-operative approach. *Journal of Clinical Oncology, 10,* 1218–1224.

Moertel, C.G., Fleming, T.R., Macdonald, J.S., Haller, D.G., Laurie, J.A., Goodman, P.J., et al. (1990). Levamisole and fluorouracil for adjuvant therapy of resected colon carcinoma. *New England Journal of Medicine, 322,* 352–358.

Moertel, C.G., Fleming, T.R., Macdonald, J.S., Haller, D.G., Laurie, J.A., Tangen, C.M., et al. (1995). Fluorouracil plus levamisole as effective adjuvant therapy after resection of stage III colon cancer: A final report. *Annals of Internal Medicine, 122,* 321–326.

National Cancer Institute. (2006). *Colon cancer PDQ®: Prevention.* Retrieved March 1, 2006, from http://www.cancer.gov/cancertopics /pdq/prevention/colon/HealthProfessional/

National Comprehensive Cancer Network. (2006a). *NCCN clinical practice guidelines in oncology: Anal canal cancer, version 2.2005.* Jenkintown, PA: Author.

National Comprehensive Cancer Network. (2006b). *NCCN clinical practice guidelines in oncology: Colon cancer, version 2.2004.* Jenkintown, PA: Author.

National Comprehensive Cancer Network. (2006c). *NCCN clinical practice guidelines in oncology: Rectal cancer, version 4.2004.* Jenkintown, PA: Author.

Nelson, H., Petrelli, N., Carlin, A., Couture, J., Fleshman, J., Guillem, J., et al. (2001). Guidelines 2000 for colon and rectal cancer surgery. *Journal of the National Cancer Institute, 93,* 583–596.

Nguyen, N., & Antoine, J. (2002). Radiation enteritis. In M. Feldman, L. Friedman, & M. Sleisenger (Eds.), *Sleisenger and Fordtran's gastrointestinal and liver disease* (7th ed., pp. 1994–2004). Philadelphia: Saunders.

Novartis Pharmaceuticals Corp. (2005). Gleevec [Package insert]. East Hanover, NJ: Author.

Pozzo, C., Basso, M., Cassano, A., Quirino, M., Schinzari, G., Trigila, N., et al. (2004). Neoadjuvant treatment of unresectable liver disease with irinotecan and 5-fluorouracil plus folinic acid in colorectal cancer patients. *Annals of Oncology, 15,* 933–939.

Raut, C., Posner, M., Desai, J., Morgan, J., George, S., Zahrieh, D., et al. (2006). Surgical management of advanced gastrointestinal stromal tumors after treatment with targeted systemic therapy using kinase inhibitors. *Journal of Clinical Oncology, 24,* 2325–2331.

Rossi, H., & Rothenberger, D. (2006). Surgical treatment of colon cancer. *Surgical Oncology Clinics of North America, 15,* 109–127.

Ryan, D., Compton, C., & Mayer, R. (2000). Carcinoma of the anal canal. *New England Journal of Medicine, 342,* 792–800.

Saif, M. (2004). Oral calcium ameliorating oxaliplatin-induced peripheral neuropathy. *Journal of Applied Research, 4,* 576–582.

Saltz, L., Cox, J., Blanke, C., Rosen, L., Fehrenbacher, L., Moore, M., et al. (2000). Irinotecan plus fluorouracil and leucovorin for metastatic colorectal cancer. *New England Journal of Medicine, 343,* 905–914.

Saltz, L., Lenz, H., Kindler, H., Hochster, H., Wadler, S., Hoff, P., et al. (2005). Interim report of randomized phase II trial of cetuximab/bevacizumab/irinotecan versus cetuximab/bevacizumab in irinotecan-refractory colorectal cancer [Abstract 169B]. *Program and abstracts of the American Society of Clinical Oncology gastrointestinal cancers symposium; January 27–29, 2005; Hollywood, FL.*

Saltz, L., Niedzwiecki, D., Hollis, D., Goldberg, R.M., Hantel, J.P., Thomas, A.L.A., et al. (2004). Irinotecan plus fluorouracil/leucovorin (IFL) versus fluorouracil/leucovorin (FL) alone in stage III colon cancer. *Journal of Clinical Oncology, 22*(Suppl. 14), 3500.

Sargent, D.J., Goldberg, R.M., Jacobson, S.D., Macdonald, J.S., Labianca, R., Haller, D.G., et al. (2001). *New England Journal of Medicine, 245,* 1091–1097.

Savage, D., & Antman, K. (2002). Imatinib mesylate—A new oral targeted therapy. *New England Journal of Medicine, 346,* 683–693.

Schrag, D., Chung, K., Flombaum, C., & Saltz, L. (2005). Cetuximab therapy and symptomatic hypomagnesemia. *Journal of the National Cancer Institute, 97,* 1221–1224.

Sengupta, S., & Tjandra, J.J. (2001). Local excision of rectal cancer: What is the evidence? *Diseases of the Colon and Rectum, 44,* 1345–1361.

Sun, W., & Haller, D. (2005). Adjuvant therapy of colon cancer. *Seminars in Oncology, 32,* 95–102.

Sweed, M., & Meropol, N. (2001). Assessment, diagnosis and staging. In D. Berg (Ed.), *Contemporary issues in colorectal cancer: A nursing perspective* (pp. 65–79). Sudbury, MA: Jones and Bartlett.

Takayama, T., Katsuki, S., Takahashi, Y., Ohi, M., Nojiri, S., Sakamaki, S., et al. (1998). Aberrant crypt foci of the colon as precursors of adenoma and cancer. *New England Journal of Medicine, 339,* 1277–1284.

Thomas, R., Quinn, M., Schuler, B., & Grem, L. (2003). Hypersensitivity and idiosyncratic reactions to oxaliplatin. *Cancer, 97,* 2301–2307.

Twelves, C., Wong, A., Nowacki, M.P., Abt, M., Burris, H., Carrato, A., et al. (2005). Capecitabine as adjuvant treatment for stage III colon cancer. *New England Journal of Medicine, 352,* 2696–2704.

U.S. Food and Drug Administration. (2006a). *Drug information pathfinder.* Bethesda, MD: Author.

U.S. Food and Drug Administration, Center for Drug Evaluation and Research. (2006b). *What's new by date.* Bethesda, MD: Author.

Van Cutsem, E., Twelves, C., Cassidy, J., Allman, D., Bajetta, E., Boyer, M., et al. (2001). Oral capecitabine compared with intravenous fluorouracil plus leucovorin in patients with metastatic colorectal cancer: Results of a large phase III study. *Journal of Clinical Oncology, 19,* 4097–4106.

Viale, P., Fung, A., & Zitella, L. (2005). Advanced colorectal cancer: Current treatment and nursing management with economic considerations. *Clinical Journal of Oncology Nursing, 9,* 541–552.

Went, P., Dirnhofer, S., Bundi, M., Mirlacher, M., Schraml, P., Mangialaio, S., et al. (2004). Prevalence of KIT expression in human tumors. *Journal of Clinical Oncology, 22,* 4514–4522.

Wilkes, G. (2005). Colon, rectal, and anal cancers. In C.H. Yarbro, M.H. Frogge, & M. Goodman (Eds.), *Cancer nursing: Principles and practice* (6th ed., pp. 1155–1214). Sudbury, MA: Jones and Bartlett.

Wilkes, G., & Barton-Burke, M. (2006). *2006 oncology nursing drug handbook.* Sudbury, MA: Jones and Bartlett.

Wolmark, N. (2005, May). *NSABP protocol C-07 firmly reinforces MOSAIC trial results in favor of oxaliplatin.* Paper presented at the American Society of Clinical Oncology, Atlanta, GA.

Wolmark, N., Fisher, B., Wieand, H.S., Henry, R.S., Lerner, H., Legault-Poisson, S., et al. (1984). The prognostic significance of preoperative carcinoembryonic antigen levels in colorectal cancer. Results from National Surgical Adjuvant Breast and Bowel Project (NSABP) clinical trials. *Annals of Surgery, 199,* 375–382.

Xiong, H.Q., & Ajani, J.A. (2004). Treatment of colorectal cancer metastasis: The role of chemotherapy. *Cancer Metastasis Reviews, 23*(1–2), 145–163.

CHAPTER 6

Nursing Care of Patients With Gastrointestinal Cancers

Joyce P. Griffin-Sobel, RN, PhD, AOCN®, APRN,BC

Introduction

Evidence-based nursing care is an essential component in caring for the patient with gastrointestinal (GI) cancer. Thorough health assessment, individualized care planning, and integration of the patient's needs at all stages of treatment are crucial for optimum quality of life. Similar presenting signs and symptoms may be seen for patients with cancers of the GI tract, and many have substantial symptomatology during treatment. This chapter will look at some of the commonalities in nursing care.

Assessment

An essential first step in assessing nursing care needs is to have a discussion with the patient and/or family who has a complaint or reason for seeking health care. Ascertain the chief complaint, history of the chief complaint, and pertinent family history. Explore the familial patterns of cancer, particularly colorectal, ovarian, and uterine cancers and melanoma. Question the patient about any substances used, including a smoking/tobacco history, alcohol intake (type and amount), and the use of any illicit drugs. Assess past medical history, the use of prescription and over-the-counter drugs, alternative treatments, and allergies. Determine the socioeconomic status of the patient, including insurance coverage. The patient's educational history also is an important factor, particularly when determining health literacy.

The patient's cultural background should be explored and incorporated, when possible, into the plan of care. Ethnicity plays a role in how a person views illness, health beliefs, communicating about disease with healthcare providers and family members, and self-care (Itano, 2005). Reviews of the literature have described African Americans as being mistrustful of the healthcare system, Hispanics and African Americans as being fatalistic about a diagnosis of cancer, and Asian/Pacific Islanders and Hispanics as regarding suffering as an inevitable part of life or as a punishment from God (Itano). However, to avoid stereotypical responses to patients, conducting a cultural assessment of the patient and family is important. Open-ended interview questions allow patients to describe, in their own words, the cultural practices that are important and relevant to their health care. Observations by the professional nurse add pertinent information to allow personalization of the cancer care experience. Ask the patient to describe his or her cultural background, specific dietary or cultural practices, how he or she would like to be addressed, and the importance of religion and spirituality in his or her life. If you meet the patient for the first time in a hospital room, notice if scriptures or other cultural and/or religious items are in plain view. If so, that is a significant statement on the importance of those items to the patient. How does the patient express pain, interact with healthcare professionals, or use body language? All of these nursing observations are important to culturally appropriate care for the patient and should be recorded.

A thorough review of symptoms is essential. Specific symptoms and questions for patients with GI disorders can be found in Figure 6-1.

Presenting Signs and Symptoms

In esophageal cancer, patients may complain of pain or difficulty swallowing, weight loss, and a feeling of a "lump" in the throat (see Figure 2-1). Persistent, progressive dysphagia and hoarseness commonly are described. Painful swallowing, or odynophagia, also may be seen. Patients with gastric cancer often have indigestion, abdominal discomfort, sensation of fullness, unexplained weight loss, and pain. Patients with colorectal cancer (CRC) may have no presenting symptoms but can have changes in stool quality or caliber. Tenesmus, or uncontrollable straining, may be found in patients with rectal cancers. Physical examination findings may include palpable masses, hepatomegaly, altered or absent bowel sounds, and altered skin turgor and texture from nutritional compromise.

Figure 6-1. Review of Patient Symptoms

Diet. Describe what you have eaten in the last 24 hours. What foods do you enjoy the most? Do you have any food intolerances? Have you had a change in the types or consistency of foods you can eat? Do you have heartburn or pain before or after eating? Do you experience diarrhea or flatulence after eating dairy products, or do you have any other signs of lactose intolerance, such as bloating, nausea, or cramping? Do you have any problems with your teeth or gums or any oral lesions?

Pain. Location, intensity, precipitating or relieving factors, and any associated symptoms

Diarrhea or constipation. Stool characteristics, nocturnal diarrhea, number of stools per day, odor, flatulence, tenesmus, blood in the stool, or other associated symptoms

General gastrointestinal symptoms. Anorexia, early satiety, feeling of fullness, dyspepsia, difficulty swallowing or pain with swallowing, feeling of a lump in the throat or foreign body sensation, weight loss or gain, or expanding abdominal girth

Medication history. Prescribed and nonprescribed treatments such as coffee enemas, herbal remedies, over-the-counter antidiarrheals or laxatives, opioids

General symptoms. Dyspnea, cough, hoarseness, skin color changes, lymph node enlargements, bleeding, anemia, jaundice, itching

Lab tests. Complete blood count with differential, electrolytes, amylase, lipase, creatinine, cholesterol, liver function tests, albumin, bilirubin

Diagnostic procedures. Tests that should be considered during the workup are chest radiograph, abdominal flat plate, upper and lower gastrointestinal series with barium, computed tomography scans, ultrasound, and rectal exams.

The abdomen may be distended, and signs of distant metastases may be found. Virchow nodes (left supraclavicular nodes seen in metastatic gastric or esophageal cancer), Blumer shelf (perirectal metastases), Sister Mary Joseph nodes (periumbilical lymphadenopathy), and Krukenberg tumor (a large ovarian mass) may be seen (Pisters, Kelsen, Powell, & Tepper, 2005). Abnormal findings may be anemia in any late-stage cancer, elevated liver function tests and elevated bilirubin with liver involvement, and an elevated carcinoembryonic antigen (CEA). CEA is a tumor marker that often is elevated in CRC. A normal CEA in a nonsmoker is < 2.5 ng/ml and is up to 5 ng/ml in smokers.

Diagnostic Tests

Patients will undergo numerous procedures to obtain an accurate diagnosis, restage the tumor during treatment, and control symptoms. Nurses can perform many of these procedures at the bedside, but it is preferable for some procedures such as endoscopy to be done in the endoscopy suite where nurses are more acquainted with use of the equipment and anticipation and prevention of complications. Many procedures are done using conscious sedation. Commonly used drugs are midazolam hydrochloride (Versed®, Roche Laboratories,

Nutley, NJ) and fentanyl. Prior to any procedure, an assessment of the patient's vital signs, level of consciousness, and appropriate lab work, especially complete blood count and clotting factors, should be performed. However, the American Society for Gastrointestinal Endoscopy has advised that routine lab testing is not necessary prior to GI endoscopy (Society of Gastrointestinal Nurses and Associates [SGNA], 2003). The length of time that a patient is permitted nothing by mouth (NPO) is controversial, as some patients (older adults, children, malnourished people) are extremely susceptible to dehydration. After the procedure, the patient may not take anything by mouth until the gag reflex has returned to prevent aspiration. Full standards of practice for endoscopic procedures, including environmental safety, infection control, and guidelines for sterilizing or disinfecting endoscopes, can be found on SGNA's Web site (www.sgna.org). Guidelines also are available for the role of the GI nurse when caring for patients under moderate or deep sedation (see Figure 6-2).

Photodynamic Therapy in Esophogeal Cancer

Photodynamic therapy, performed with an esophagogastroduodenoscopy (EGD), is a procedure for patients with Barrett's esophagus, early esophageal cancer, or obstructive esophageal lesions and for recurrent or persistent lesions. It also is being used for treatment of Barrett's esophagus, psoriasis, and cutaneous cancers. A photoactive drug, porfimer sodium (Photofrin®, Axcan Pharma, Birmingham, AL) (one activated by light), is administered intravenously to a patient 40–50 hours prior to use of a KTP laser, which targets cancer cells. For esophageal lesions, a fiberoptic probe is used to deliver the laser light during an endoscopy. The procedure lasts about an hour, and the patient may have a repeat endoscopy five days later for debridement. The patient must not have had radiation therapy for four weeks prior to the procedure and will remain photosensitive for 30 days afterward, particularly the skin and eyes. Sunscreen offers no protection. It is essential that the patient comply with strict photosensitive precautions, which include

1. Wear a long-sleeved shirt, a dark-colored jacket, and long pants when outside.
2. Wear sunglasses with maximum ultraviolet light protection when outside.
3. Wear gloves and a hat with a brim to cover the ears and forehead when outside.
4. When inside, do not sit directly under a reading lamp and do not sit near a bright unshaded window (National Cancer Institute, 2004).

LASER (Light Amplification by Stimulated Emission of Radiation) is used for coagulation or vaporization of tumors of the esophagus, stomach, and colon. Lasers that are used in endoscopic procedures are the argon laser and the Nd: YAG (neodymium-yttrium-aluminum-garnet) laser. The laser transmits light energy through a quartz fiber catheter that is passed through an endoscope. These procedures are done on

Figure 6-2. Position Statement: ASGE/SGNA Role of Gastrointestinal Registered Nurses in the Management of Patients Undergoing Sedated Procedures

Disclaimer

The ASGE and SGNA assume no responsibility for the practices or recommendations of any member or other practitioner, or for the policies and practices of any practice setting. The Registered Nurse functions within the limits of state licensure, state nurse practice act, and institutional policies.

The safety and efficacy of sedation for GI procedures requires cooperation between the physician endoscopist and the GI registered nurse assistants. This statement is meant to clarify the roles of the physician and registered nurse for the safe administration of sedatives, patient monitoring during sedation, and management of sedation-related complications. In all cases, care must be provided in adherence to locally defined or state-mandated nursing scope of practice. Specific guidelines on the use of moderate[1] and deep sedation[2] have been previously published.

All patients undergoing endoscopic procedures require pre-procedural evaluation to assess their risk and to help manage problems related to pre-existing medical conditions. This assessment includes obtaining a history and performing a focused physical examination, reviewing current medications and drug allergies, assessing cardiopulmonary status, and assessing the airway, particularly if deep sedation will be used.[3] The GI nurse may assist in this assessment, however, it is the responsibility of the physician to determine the suitability of the patient for sedation.

Once the suitability of the patient for sedation has been determined, a sedation plan is formulated. This plan determines the medications to be given and the intended level of sedation. The nurse then prepares and administers the medications under the direct order and supervision of the physician. The physician may also administer medications to the patient.

During the procedure, it is the responsibility of the nurse to monitor the patient's vital signs, comfort and clinical status. The nurse records these data prior to, at intervals during, and following the procedure. The purpose of patient monitoring is to detect potential intra-procedure complications, especially those due to sedation. During endoscopy under moderate sedation, the nurse may perform interruptible tasks such as assisting with biopsy or polypectomy. For deep sedation, the registered nurse performing the patient monitoring should have no other responsibilities.[3,4] Effective communication is of paramount importance to ensure a safe and comfortable procedure.

Complications due to sedatives, although infrequent, are the most common type of complication seen during endoscopic procedures.[5] Sedatives may cause cardiopulmonary compromise and other complications such as allergic reactions, interactions with other drugs, and idiosyncratic or dose-related adverse events.[1] If these complications are recognized the physician must be promptly informed. Management of any complication that may occur is ultimately the responsibility of the physician. This may range from administration of medications to the patient (e.g., oxygen, sedative-reversal agents) to opening the airway and providing assisted ventilation (e.g., bag-mask ventilation, endotracheal intubation). The physician must be immediately available to manage complications, from the beginning of sedation until the patient has adequately recovered from their effects.

Post-procedural care should be delivered according to established protocols or written physician orders regarding the level of monitoring and discharge criteria.

Each endoscopy unit must have policies regarding the use of sedation. These policies specify the responsibilities of each member of the sedation team. Adequate training of physicians and nurses must be undertaken prior to using sedation for GI procedures. This training includes pre-procedural assessment, levels of sedation, pharmacology of sedative and reversal agents, basic life support, establishing and maintaining an adequate airway, recording vital signs and medications used, patient monitoring, and the recognition of complications.[6,7] For deep sedation, additional training with emphasis on advanced airway management and treatment of cardiovascular complications, particularly hypotension, is required. The endoscopy unit must also provide continuing education with ongoing competencies for administering and monitoring all levels of sedation, and have a functioning quality improvement assurance program.[8]

[1] Waring JP, Baron TH, Goldstein JL, Jacobson BC, Leighton JA, Mallery JS et al. Guidelines for Conscious Sedation and Monitoring during Gastrointestinal Endoscopy. Gastrointest Endosc 2003; in press.
[2] Faigel DO, Baron TH, Goldstein JL, Hirota WK, Jacobson BC, Johanson JF, et al. Guidelines for the use of deep sedation and analgesia for GI endoscopy. Gastrointest Endosc_2002;56(5):613-7.
[3] Gross JB, Bailey PL, Connis RT, Cote CJ, Davis FG, Epstein BS et al. Practice Guidelines for sedation and analgesia by non-anesthesiologists. Anesthesiology2002; 96:1004-17.
[4] Statement on Minimal Registered Nurse Staffing for Patient Care in the Endoscopy Unit: May,2002: Society of Gastroenterology Nurses and Associates' Practice Committee
[5] Eisen GM, Baron TH, Dominitz JA, Faigel DO, Goldstein JL, Johanson JF et al. Complications of upper GI endoscopy. Gastrointest Endosc 2002;55:784-93.
[6] Guidelines for training in patient monitoring and sedation and analgesia. Gastrointest Endosc 1998;48:669-71.
[7] Guidelines For Nursing Care of the Patient Receiving Sedation and Analgesia in the Gastrointestinal Endoscopy Setting : 2000: Society of Gastroenterology Nurses and Associates' Practice Committee.
[8] Establishment of gastrointestinal endoscopy areas. Gastrointest Endosc 1999;50:910-12.

Note. Copyright 2004 by the American Society of Gastrointestinal Endoscopy. Reprinted with permission.

an ambulatory basis, and precautions and nursing implications are the same as those for EGD.

Endoscopic Procedures for the Gastrointestinal Tract

Biopsies can be performed during many of these procedures. Biopsy forceps can be used in conjunction with many endoscopes, and electrocoagulating, or hot, biopsy forceps are used to coagulate tissue when bleeding is a risk (SGNA, 2003). Endoscopic biopsies can be performed in the esophagus, stomach, and small and large bowel. Endoscopic ultrasound procedures are sensitive methods of detecting malignancies. Percutaneous liver biopsy can be performed at the bedside for evaluation of jaundice, hepatitis, malignancy, or other pathologies (e.g., cirrhosis, Wilson disease, lymphoma staging, hemochromatosis). After this procedure, the patient lies on his or her right side against a sandbag and maintains that position for two hours, with strict bed rest for the next six to eight hours to prevent hematoma formation or bleeding in the liver (SGNA, 2003). Prior to the procedure, clotting parameters will be assessed, and the patient should avoid aspirin, ibuprofen, and anticoagulants for a week, depending on the physician's specifications. The patient will be NPO for eight hours prior to the procedure (National Institute of Diabetes and Digestive and Kidney Diseases, 2004).

Complications that may occur during GI procedures include perforation of the GI tract, hemorrhage, and shock. Perforation can result from trauma during the procedure or after dilatation of strictures in the esophagus resulting from radiation therapy or malignancy. Gastric perforation can result from ulcer disease. Colonic perforation can result after removal of large polyps, laser therapy, or use of excessive current (electrocautery). Signs of upper GI perforation include pain, especially in the neck area, and dysphagia. Surgical repair may be indicated. Lower GI perforations also are notable for significant complaints of pain, abdominal distention, increased tympany, and rectal drainage (SGNA, 2003). Hematemesis, hypotension, tachycardia, melena, weakness, abdominal pain, or distention may indicate GI bleeding. Rapid assessment, accompanied by interventions to maintain the airway, establish adequate fluid volume, stabilize the patient, and stop the bleeding, is a priority nursing action (see Table 6-1). Complications from a liver biopsy include hemorrhage, peritonitis, infection, or liver laceration. Observe the patient for changes in vital signs, prolonged pain radiating to the shoulder or back, or abdominal distention (SGNA, 1998).

Diagnostic procedures for the colon include colonoscopy and sigmoidoscopy. For sigmoidoscopy, the patient usually is restricted to a liquid diet for 12–24 hours and usually will be asked to self-administer an enema the night before the procedure. The patient does not need to be NPO. Flexible sigmoidoscopy is well tolerated when performed by a skilled professional, and its brief duration requires no sedation. The risk of complications, such as bleeding or perforation, is very small. The restricted area of the colon that is accessible by sigmoidoscopy, however, limits its usefulness in colorectal screening (Ransohoff & Sandler, 2002).

More than 90% of colon polyps are detected during colonoscopy (Ransohoff & Sandler, 2002). For a colonoscopy, the patient may be restricted to a liquid diet for one to three days. Thorough bowel preparations are very important, as poor preparations often lead to a failed procedure, with the patient having to undergo a second colonoscopy (Reilly & Walker, 2004). Bowel preparations in wide use currently include oral intake of a 4–6 L polyethylene glycol solution (GoLytely®, Braintree Laboratories, Braintree, MA), sometimes followed by a tap water enema, or a hyperosmotic preparation of Fleet® Phospho-soda® (Fleet Laboratories, Lynchburg, VA) or oral sodium phosphate solution. The polyethylene glycol solutions are intended to lavage the bowel, so they should be ingested over a two-hour period. Using a powdered soft drink mix, such as Crystal Light® (Kraft, Northfield, IL), makes the solution more palatable for most patients. The Phospho-soda preparation is for young, healthy people, as the circulatory system absorbs the solution. It should not be used in patients with renal, cardiac, or hepatic disease. Visicol® (Salix Pharmaceuticals, Morrisville, NC) is Fleet Phospho-soda in tablet form. Patient and physician preference, ease of completion, and cleansing efficacy influence the choice of a bowel preparation. Both methods are effective, but the oral sodium phosphate solution may be better tolerated (American Society for Gastrointestinal Endoscopy, 2001). Side effects and complications include dehydration, asymptomatic hyperphosphatemia, and hypokalemia. Nurses should encourage patients to drink fluids liberally prior to their procedure (McCormick, Kibbe, & Morgan, 2002).

Biopsies and the removal of polyps are performed during colonoscopy; polyps are removed with wire snares or hot biopsy forceps. The nurse in the GI lab usually opens and closes the forceps. The electrosurgical unit is a generator that produces a high-frequency current for cutting and coagulation, both of which are used to transect the polyp from the mucosa. Polypectomies include

- Complete excisions using biopsy forceps and ablation with a coagulation current if the polyp is a small (< 8 mm in diameter) sessile (attached to mucosa on a broad base) polyp.
- Sessile polyps < 1 cm in diameter are removed with a snare and cautery.
- Pedunculated (attached to colon mucosa via a stalk) polyps are snared and transected using cautery.
- Larger polyps are removed after segmental resection.

Bleeding is the most common complication, along with adverse reactions to sedation and, rarely, perforation. Nurses assisting with the procedure carefully monitor the patient for changes in vital signs, diaphoresis, cold clammy skin, abdominal distention, and signs of bleeding (SGNA, 1998).

Table 6-1. Gastrointestinal Procedures

Procedure	Purpose	Patient Teaching	Nursing Implications
Esophagogastroduodenoscopy (EGD); endoscopic procedure	Directly visualize the esophagus, stomach, and duodenum	Patient is nothing by mouth (NPO) for two to eight hours, depending on institutional policy and procedure. Throat will be anesthetized; may not eat or drink until gag reflex returns. Conscious sedation may be used.	Complications include hemorrhage and perforation. Observe the patient for significant pain, bleeding, dyspnea, hemoptysis, and change in vital signs.
Esophageal dilation with bougienage or hydrostatic balloons; endoscopic procedure	To dilate the esophagus to facilitate swallowing in patients with lesions or strictures of the esophagus	Conscious sedation will be used. Patient is NPO for six to eight hours prior to procedure, and no foods or fluids by mouth until gag reflex returns.	Bougienage is dilation with bougies, or soft rubber weighted dilators of varying sizes. Dilation often is accompanied by stent placement. Complications include hemorrhage and perforation.
Esophageal stent placement; usually done in conjunction with EGD	Palliative treatment for obstructing esophageal lesions and strictures	Patient NPO for six to eight hours before the procedure and until gag reflex returns. Wire mesh stent placed over a guidewire endoscopically; permanent device inserted to expand the lumen of the esophagus	Observe for hemorrhage, airway compromise, and signs of perforation (e.g., pain, bleeding, changes in vital signs).
Endoscopic retrograde cholangiopancreatography	Endoscopic procedure to visualize biliary and pancreatic ducts	NPO for six to eight hours before the procedure and until gag reflex returns	Usually done to evaluate a patient with jaundice and to locate stones or tumor within the biliary tract. Pancreatitis is a complication. Observe for pain, bleeding, and airway compromise.
Flexible sigmoidoscopy	Procedure to visualize the rectum and sigmoid and distal descending colon up to 65 cm	Bowel prep of an enema the night before is necessary. Procedure is uncomfortable. No sedation typically is used.	Ensure patient has been adequately prepped. Complications include perforation and pain. Can be done by an RN with appropriate training.*
Colonoscopy	Procedure to visualize the entire colon to the ileocecal valve. Polyps can be removed and biopsied using this technique.	Adequate bowel prep with polyethylene glycol or sodium phosphate is essential. Conscious sedation is used.	Assess patient for signs of dehydration. Complications include infection or perforation.

Note. Based on information from Society of Gastroenterology Nurses and Associates, 2001, 2003. *For the Society of Gastroenterology Nurses and Associates position statement on the "Performance of Flexible Sigmoidoscopy by Registered Nurses for the Purpose of Colorectal Cancer Screening," visit http://www.sgna.org/Resources/guidelines/guideline1.cfm.

Surgical Nursing Care

Curative treatment for GI cancers often is surgical. Palliative surgery, such as stenting, is less extensive and can add significantly to quality of life (see Figure 6-3).

Surgery for Esophageal Cancer

Surgical resection of the esophagus is the preferred treatment for localized tumors of the esophagus. Patients with unresectable disease can be palliated with nonsurgical therapies, such as stenting. Outcomes after esophagectomy are directly related to both surgeon and hospital volume (Posner, Forastiere, & Minsky, 2005). Stage I–III cancers are potentially resectable. Surgeon preference and tumor and patient characteristics help determine the optimal surgery. Esophagogastrectomy can be accomplished in two ways: the transthoracic, which uses abdominal and right thoracic incisions and creates an anastomosis at the upper thorax (Ivor-Lewis technique), or neck, or the transhiatal technique, which uses

Figure 6-3. Expandable Metal Stents for the Treatment of Cancerous Obstructions of the Gastrointestinal Tract

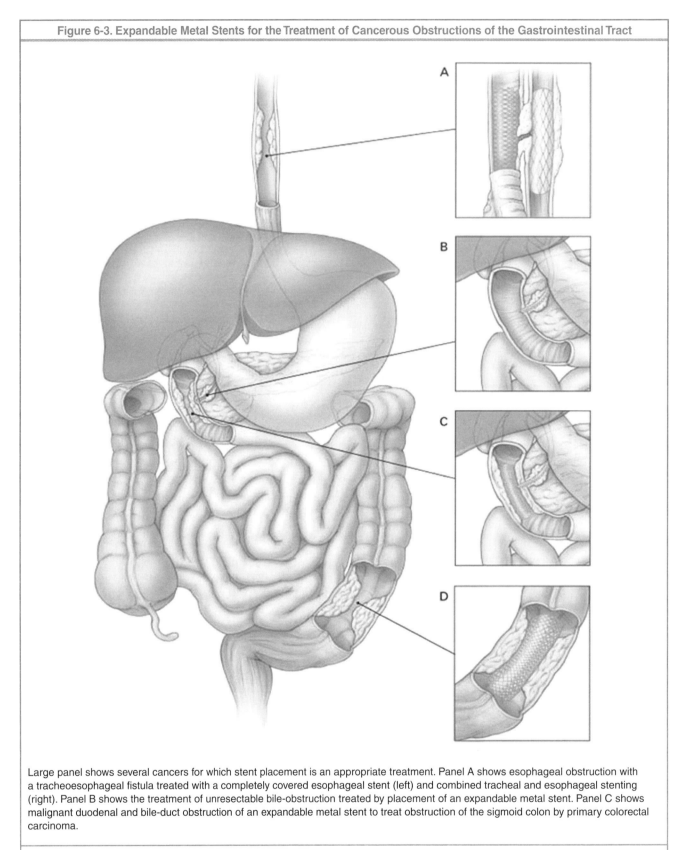

Large panel shows several cancers for which stent placement is an appropriate treatment. Panel A shows esophageal obstruction with a tracheoesophageal fistula treated with a completely covered esophageal stent (left) and combined tracheal and esophageal stenting (right). Panel B shows the treatment of unresectable bile-obstruction treated by placement of an expandable metal stent. Panel C shows malignant duodenal and bile-duct obstruction of an expandable metal stent to treat obstruction of the sigmoid colon by primary colorectal carcinoma.

abdominal and left cervical incisions. Both methods use the stomach to replace the esophagus (National Comprehensive Cancer Network [NCCN], 2006b).

The transhiatal esophagectomy is gaining increasing favor because of the rising incidence of adenocarcinoma of the distal esophagus, which is effectively resected via this method (Posner et al., 2005). The majority of the esophagus is removed, and the gastric fundus is pulled up into the mediastinum and anastomosed to the cervical esophagus (Tsottles & Reedy, 2005). A shorter operation is necessary, but the incidence of anastomotic leak is higher than with other techniques. The Ivor-Lewis procedure involves resecting the esophagus and stomach, which is pulled up to anastomose with the esophageal stump at the cervical or intrathoracic level (Tsottles & Reedy). The transthoracic approach allows a wider dissection, but evidence does not favor one technique over another, although the transhiatal approach has a lower rate of complications (Enzinger & Mayer, 2003; Posner et al.). Trials evaluating the impact of preoperative chemoradiotherapy may improve patient outcomes after esophageal surgeries.

Complications include respiratory compromise, leak at the anastomosis, and wound infection. Aggressive pulmonary toilet with frequent turning, coughing and deep breathing, use of incentive spirometry, and physical therapy are necessary. Monitor fluid balance closely, as overhydration can contribute to respiratory compromise. Observe all wounds and tubes for signs of infection or bleeding. Dilatations of the esophagus because of strictures often are required postoperatively. Nutrition is a concern for any patient having esophageal surgery, and a nutritionist should be consulted early in the process (see Table 6-2). Patients often experience early satiety, gastric stasis, and

dumping syndrome from the rapid passage of food through the GI tract because of the lack of an esophagus (Tsottles & Reedy, 2005) (see Table 6-3).

Surgery for Cancer of the Stomach

Resection of cancers of the stomach is the only curative treatment available, as described in Chapter 4. Total gastrectomy, with or without extensive lymphadenectomy, or subtotal gastrectomy, for patients who cannot undergo the more radical procedure, are the surgeries performed most often. Subtotal gastrectomy has equivalent results with fewer side effects compared to total gastrectomy for distal cancers of the stomach (NCCN, 2006c) (see Table 6-4). Total gastrectomy involves excising the stomach and part of the esophagus and duodenum, with the jejunum anastomosed to the esophagus. A Roux-en-Y jejunostomy allows biliary secretion drainage (O'Connor, 2005). Subtotal gastrectomy involves removal of the pyloric portion of the stomach with anastomosis to the duodenum (gastroduodenostomy or Billroth I) or anastomosis to the jejunum (gastrojejunostomy or Billroth II) (Grzelak, 2004). Billroth I procedures are more limited resections and have a lower cure rate (O'Connor).

Postoperative care involves routine nursing observations for changes in fluid and electrolytes, respiratory compromise, bleeding, and infection. Additional complications include anastomotic leak, reflux aspiration, and nutritional compromise. Weight loss is a common complication, and a nutritionist should be involved in the patient's care. Enteral feeding or hyperalimentation may be necessary. Postprandial dumping syndrome is a commonly reported symptom after

Table 6-2. Special Considerations for Nutrition for Patients Who Have Had an Esophagectomy		
Treatment	**Diet Upgrade in Hospital**	**Diet Upgrade After Discharge**
Esophagectomy	Usually nothing by mouth until postoperative day four On day four, a clear liquid diet, as well as an isotonic feeding, is started. Tube feedings are cycled to night feedings to free the patient through the day and to encourage increased oral intake. The patient may be on tube feedings from two to four weeks. By postoperative day seven or eight, the patient's diet is increased to a full liquid diet. By two to four weeks after surgery, tube feeds will be decreased as soft foods are tolerated.	Suggest two ounces of clear liquids every two hours, and increase until the patient is able to tolerate six ounces every four hours. Continue this schedule as the patient goes to full liquids. Encourage the patient to avoid carbonated soft drinks the first six to eight weeks after surgery. Encourage the patient to drink nutritional supplements several times per day if unable to eat enough regular foods to meet his or her nutritional needs. Avoid dairy products such as milk, cottage cheese, and pudding, as these may cause diarrhea. Encourage small, frequent meals throughout the day. Recommend that the patient sit up straight for one to two hours after each meal. Tell the patient to avoid sweets such as pies, cookies, and pastries that may cause diarrhea or dumping syndrome. Avoid foods that are spicy and gas forming to eliminate gastrointestinal distress.

Note. From "Esophageal and Gastric Cancers" (p. 54), by K. Masino in V.J. Kogut and S.L. Luthringer (Eds.), *Nutritional Issues in Cancer Care*, 2005, Pittsburgh, PA: Oncology Nursing Society. Copyright 2005 by the Oncology Nursing Society. Reprinted with permission.

Table 6-3. Common Side Effects of Esophageal Cancer Treatment, Causes, and Management

Side Effect	Possible Causes	Management
Difficulty or painful swallowing	Tumor location Inflammation/pain in esophagus because of endoscopic surgery, radiation, or chemotherapy Anastomotic stricture after esophagectomy Tumor recurrence Tumor ingrowth in stent	Encourage small, frequent, soft, moist meals and snacks. Encourage patient to drink high-calorie liquid nutritional supplements several times per day if patient is unable to eat enough regular foods to meet his or her nutritional needs. Insert feeding tube if patient is unable to drink and eat sufficient calories to maintain his or her weight.
Early satiety, anorexia, and weight loss	Tumor location, surgical treatment, chemotherapy, and radiation	Encourage small, frequent meals. Encourage patient to consume high-calorie foods such as ice cream, puddings, cheeses, milkshakes, cream soups, eggs, and lunchmeats and spreads, such as tuna and chicken. Limit fluids with meals, but encourage patient to sip fluids throughout the day to meet fluid intake needs. Augment meals with liquid supplements. Patients who have had an esophagectomy must drink slowly to decrease chance of dumping syndrome. Provide appetite stimulants. Cycle or decrease tube feeds to help to increase oral intake.
Gas bloating	Altered anatomy	Use antiflatuence medication, such as simethicone. Encourage small, frequent meals.
Reflux, regurgitation, and esophagitis	Removal of distal esophageal sphincter with esophagectomy Stents and lasers placed at the gastroesophageal junction Increased incidence of heartburn	Follow antireflux diet (i.e., no citrus, tomato, fatty foods, coffee, or chocolate). Encourage small, frequent meals. Encourage patient to stand up or walk after eating. Elevate head of bed 30°–45° during times of rest or bedtime, especially if patient is receiving tube feedings. Use antireflux medications if needed. Try aloe vera liquid before meals.
Dumping syndrome and diarrhea	Occurs in patients who have had an esophagectomy secondary to removal of the distal esophageal sphincter Symptoms that may occur 15–60 minutes after a meal include nausea, vomiting, diarrhea, dizziness, and palpitations. Tube feeding intolerance Infectious diarrhea	Encourage small, frequent meals. Avoid lactose in diet. Avoid large amounts of concentrated sweets. Eat dry meals with fluids consumed 30 minutes after meals. Change tube feeding formula if not tolerated. Begin standard antidiarrheal medications. Use medication if infectious diarrhea is present. Try probiotics, such as Lactinex®, or yogurt. Encourage patient to eat a low-fat and low-roughage diet. Encourage increased fluid intake; patient may need IV hydration.
Constipation	Both pain and antinausea medications have a constipating effect. Changes in eating habits or eating a decreased amount Decreased physical activity Decreased fluid intake	Encourage patient to use laxatives and stool softeners as directed. Encourage patient to eat at the same times every day. Encourage patient to drink 8–10 cups of liquid each day, including water, prune juice, and warm liquids. Encourage patient to eat more high-fiber foods. Begin bowel program with stool softeners and laxatives, as needed.
Anastomotic leak	Surgical complication after an esophagectomy (food may be seen leaking out of neck incision)	Nothing by mouth as determined by physician (may be a three- to four-week time period). Begin full nutritional support with jejunal feeds. Retry oral diet as determined by physician.
Chyle leak	Thoracic duct is accidentally nicked during surgery.	Try a very low-fat diet (less than 10 grams) to include flat soft drinks, juices, and broths. Use tube feedings that are semi-elemental and high in MCT oils. Use total parenteral nutrition if drainage persists with the above recommendations. Somatostatin may be of benefit once leak is determined.

Note. From "Esophageal and Gastric Cancers" (pp. 51–52), by K. Masino in V.J. Kogut and S.L. Luthringer (Eds.), *Nutritional Issues in Cancer Care*, 2005, Pittsburgh, PA: Oncology Nursing Society. Copyright 2005 by the Oncology Nursing Society. Reprinted with permission.

gastric surgeries, and the patient should be instructed to eat smaller meals and to refrain from fluid intake during meals to slow down digestion.

Patients also may develop anemia from deficiencies of vitamin B_{12} or folate, the former occurring from loss of parietal cells in the stomach. Assess the patient for dysphagia or gastric retention, both of which can develop after vagotomy and contribute to the patient's nutritional compromise. Pain control, as with all surgeries, is an essential component of excellent postoperative care.

Complications include respiratory compromise, leaks at the anastomosis site, infection, esophagitis, and bleeding. Nutrition-al concerns postoperatively are a significant problem. Patients may become anemic from B_{12} or folate deficiencies because of reduced gastric acid secretions. Dumping syndrome often is a significant problem, and the measures found in Table 6-4 should be reviewed with the patient and family (O'Connor, 2005).

Surgery for Cancer of the Colon, Rectum, or Anus

Surgeries for the colon, rectum, and anus have been previously described. The trend in surgery is to minimize the

Table 6-4. Common Side Effects of Gastric Cancer Treatment, Causes, and Management

Side Effect	Possible Causes	Management
Anemia	Decreased vitamin B_{12} absorption because of loss of intrinsic factor secondary to a total gastrectomy Decreased iron absorption from either a partial or a total gastrectomy. This can be a late complication of a gastrectomy. A folate deficiency may occur secondary to malabsorption.	Patient will need vitamin B_{12} levels measured at baseline and then every three months afterward. In a mild deficiency, may try oral vitamin B_{12}. In a severe deficiency, patient will require vitamin B_{12} internally. Patient will require iron supplementation for about four to six months if a deficiency is present. Patient will require a multivitamin with folate to prevent a deficiency.
Fat malabsorption	Increased transit time that prevents sufficient mixing of food with digestive enzymes Decreased enzyme production	Encourage patient to try a low-fat diet. Patient may need to use medium-chain triglycerides if steatorrhea is present. Patient may need pancreatic enzymes. Fat-soluble vitamins may need to be added to patient's diet.
Lactose intolerance	May occur despite intact jejunum	Encourage patient to try a low-fat diet. Encourage patient to use lactase enzymes.
Metabolic bone disease	Metabolic bone disease can be seen as a late complication after a gastrectomy. This may be caused by malabsorption of fat-soluble vitamins, including vitamin D, and poor food and lactose intake. Patients also may have decreased calcium metabolism.	Patients will need vitamin D and calcium supplementation in addition to a daily multivitamin.
Delayed gastric emptying	Patients with truncal vagotomy may have a higher incidence. Symptoms include discomfort or bloating that may last a few hours and possibly emesis.	Encourage smaller and more frequent meals. Patient may need a prokinetic agent.
Reactive hypoglycemia	Can be the result of late dumping syndrome Late dumping is caused by a quick rise and then fall of blood sugars secondary to increased insulin. Can occur one to three hours after a meal and cause symptoms of sweating, palpitations, and fatigue	Encourage smaller and more frequent protein-dense meals. Tell patient to avoid large amounts of concentrated sweets.

Note. From "Esophageal and Gastric Cancers" (pp. 58–59), by K. Masino in V.J. Kogut and S.L. Luthringer (Eds.), *Nutritional Issues in Cancer Care*, 2005, Pittsburgh, PA: Oncology Nursing Society. Copyright 2005 by the Oncology Nursing Society. Reprinted with permission.

amount of resection using preoperative chemotherapy and/or radiotherapy. In colon resections, a minimum of 12 nodes should be examined, and laparoscopic-assisted colorectal procedures can be considered if the tumor meets minimum requirements and the surgeon has the appropriate experience. Rectal tumors can be resected transanally if the tumor is small; via an abdominoperineal resection, necessitating a colostomy; or via a low anterior resection or coloanal anastomosis. Anal carcinomas, after the patient has preoperative chemotherapy and radiotherapy, can be resected with low anterior resections (NCCN, 2006a) (see Table 6-5).

Nursing interventions for major surgical procedures are undergoing some rethinking, particularly the preoperative procedures that routinely have been instituted. Despite the increasing attention that nurses are paying to patients' nutritional status, current evidence about preoperative nutrition continues to be neglected. In 1999, the American Society of Anesthesiologists (ASA) Task Force on Preoperative Fasting developed evidence-based guidelines on preoperative fasting. These guidelines noted that pulmonary aspiration is rare, little relationship exists between fasting duration and gastric contents, prolonged fasting can be associated with significant adverse effects, and clear liquids leave the stomach immediately after ingestion (ASA, 1999). The guidelines allow for ingestion of clear liquids up to two hours before elective surgery requiring general, regional, or sedation anesthesia, with a light breakfast permitted six hours before the procedure. Eight hours should elapse between a heavy meal and surgery.

Crenshaw and Winslow (2002) conducted a descriptive study to ascertain compliance with the revised ASA guidelines. They interviewed 155 patients who had undergone elective, nonobstetric, nongastrointestinal surgery. Findings were surprising: Patients had fasted from liquids and solids an average of 12 hours, with some patients fasting for 20 hours. Most patients (91%) were instructed to maintain NPO after midnight, even when surgeries were scheduled for late afternoon. Sixty-three percent of patients had received preoperative instruction from a nurse. Even more concerning, 58% of the patients were taking significant medications (anticoagulants, diabetic medications, oral contraceptives, cardiac or seizure medications), and 22% had received no instruction about their medications, whereas others had varying instructions to take or not. Patients reported significant levels of thirst, hunger, and worry.

This study demonstrated little change in practice in response to the revised ASA guidelines. It is concerning that the adverse effects of fasting, including thirst, hunger, irritability, headache, dehydration, and hypoglycemia, did not outweigh the inconvenience of departing from tradition or the exaggerated concern about aspiration. Nurses have an obligation to collaborate with physicians to discuss appropriate preoperative fasting instructions and to implement hospital policy. This study should be extended to nonelective and GI surgery patients.

Another preoperative routine for elective colorectal surgery is mechanical bowel preparation, involving the use of polyethylene glycol solutions or sodium phosphate solutions the day before surgery, along with a clear liquid diet the day before surgery. The purpose of these procedures was to minimize the risk of infection or fecal contamination of the operative field. However, a recent meta-analysis of patients (N = 1,592) undergoing low anterior resections found no difference in wound infections, anastomotic leakage, or mortality among patients having a mechanical bowel preparation and those who did not. More patients who had the mechanical bowel preparation experienced peritonitis (Guenaga, Matos, Castro, Atallah, & Wille-Jorgensen, 2005). Two other meta-analyses revealed similar results, but the incidence of anastomotic leakage was higher in the mechanical preparation groups (Bucher, Mermillod, Morel, & Soravia, 2004; Slim, Vicaut, Panis, & Chipponi, 2004). Direct clinical evidence demonstrates no benefit from mechanical bowel preparations compared to no preparations. A higher incidence of anastomotic leakage was seen in patients having a bowel preparation, and serious adverse side effects, such as hyponatremia and seizures, can occur after oral sodium phosphate preparations (Gray & Colwell, 2005).

Some traditions of postoperative care also are being questioned. Many nursing textbooks recommend that nurses assess postoperative bowel sounds for 20 minutes—5 minutes per quadrant. Many nurses do not comply with this recommendation. One team (Madsen et al., 2005) used the Iowa Model of Evidence-Based Practice to promote quality care and examined the practices of auscultating bowel sounds postoperatively. They noted the scarcity of current research on the topic. The return of GI motility after abdominal surgery begins with random electrical impulses, progressing to coordinated muscular activity and propulsion. Motility is seen in the small intestine in 4–24 hours and in the colon 3–7 days postoperatively. Auscultation of the abdomen in the early postoperative period is not an accurate method of assessing bowel activity because early sounds are probably small intestine contractions. The team developed a practice guideline and implemented and evaluated it. Findings revealed that clinical signs other than bowel sounds, such as the return of flatus and the first bowel movement postoperatively, are more appropriate assessment criteria for the return of bowel function. Other assessment criteria are to assess the patient for presence or absence of abdominal pain or discomfort, feeling bloated, or feeling hungry. This project was a reminder of how many "traditional" nursing practices are not scientifically based and should be questioned.

Ostomy Surgery

For patients who require an ostomy, preoperative teaching is extremely important. If the creation of the ostomy is elective, teaching on the procedure itself, wound care, dietary

Table 6-5. Surgical Interventions for Colon, Rectal, and Anal Cancers

Surgery	Details	Risks	Complications	Nursing Care
Curative radical colectomy	Section of colon with *en bloc* resection of adjacent mesentery	Hemorrhage, infection, leak at anastomosis	Deep vein thromboses, infection, aspiration, paralytic ileus, inadequate nutrition	Pain control, preventing respiratory complications, wound care, promoting bowel function with early ambulation
Standard colectomy with lymphadenectomy	Minimum of 5–10 cm on either side of colon cancer is resected	Hemorrhage, infection, anastomotic leak, dehiscence of wound	Deep vein thromboses, infection, aspiration, paralytic ileus, inadequate nutrition	Pain control, preventing respiratory complications, wound care, promoting bowel function with early ambulation
Laparoscopic colectomy	For localized tumors where resection and anastomosis are performed	May be necessary to go to open procedure	Deep vein thromboses, infection, aspiration, paralytic ileus, inadequate nutrition	Pain control, preventing respiratory complications, wound care, promoting bowel function with early ambulation
Colonic stenting	Palliation for malignant obstructions	–	Deep vein thromboses, infection, aspiration, paralytic ileus, inadequate nutrition	Pain control, preventing respiratory complications
Transanal excision of rectal tumor	Local excision of anal tumor	–	Urinary retention, mild pain, hemorrhage	Pain control, preventing respiratory complications, wound care, promoting bowel function with early ambulation
Low anterior resection of rectum and distal colon	Rectal or distal colon lesions for tumors located 6–15 cm from the anal verge	Removal of descending colon, to lower one-third of rectum	Dehiscence, bowel ischemia	Pain control, preventing respiratory complications, wound care, promoting bowel function with early ambulation
Total mesorectal excision The mesorectum contains the blood supply and lymphatics of the rectum, and most involved lymph nodes of rectal cancer are there.	Coloanal anastomosis and creation of intestinal pouches can be employed to maintain anal sphincters.	–	Dehiscence, bowel ischemia	Pain control, preventing respiratory complications, wound care, promoting bowel function with early ambulation
Abdominoperineal resection for distal colon and rectal cancers	Permanent colostomy created Removal of sigmoid colon and rectum with abdominal and perineal incisions	–	Deep vein thromboses, infection, aspiration, paralytic ileus, inadequate nutrition	Pain control, preventing respiratory complications, wound care, promoting bowel function with early ambulation

Note. Based on information from Perretta et al., 2006; Rossi & Rothenberger, 2006; Wilkes, 2005.

restrictions (see Figure 6-4), and pain management postoperatively should be given. Arranging a visit with a person living with an ostomy is a successful method of allaying anxiety for the patient. Groups such as the United Ostomy Association can be contacted to assist with such visits.

Stoma site selection is critical to quality of life in a person with an ostomy, and the patient should be seen by a wound, ostomy, and continence nurse (WOCN) or enterostomal therapist for site placement of the stoma (sitting a stoma). The specialist evaluates the patient in several different positions to note folds, muscle movement, and creases. This is particularly important for a patient with an obese abdomen, as there can be large shifts of tissue when the person changes positions. The WOCN may mark more than one stoma site, as the location of the stoma may need to change once the surgeon enters the abdomen (Colwell & Fichera, 2005).

After the patient returns from surgery, the dressing is closely monitored for signs of bleeding. Vital signs are monitored, and the patient is observed for signs of infection. The stoma should be pink or red with a small amount of oozing. The stoma will begin to function approximately three days after surgery. The oncology nurse and the enterostomal therapy nurse can jointly plan on a teaching schedule and gradual assumption of self-care by the patient. Skin care for the peristomal skin should be emphasized to the patient, because irritation under the appliance will affect its adherence. The patient should be taught to wash the skin with a mild soap and water, while using a tampon or rolled gauze in the orifice of the stoma to control drainage. Dry the area by patting, and apply the peristomal skin barrier, which may be a wafer or paste. If irritation is present, applying karaya powder can alleviate discomfort. The appliance is attached to the skin barrier. The patient should empty the pouch on regular intervals so the appliance does not pull off because of the weight of the contents.

Emotional support must be provided, as patients may have significant changes in body image and lifestyle. The patient should be taught about the anatomic changes that occur because of surgery and care of the stoma. Teaching during stressful times should be simplistic and repetitive, with illustrations and written instructions provided for the patient and family to peruse. Sexuality issues need to be discussed openly with the patient, including the use of alternative positions that may be more comfortable (Manning, 2004).

Communication

Striving to ensure that communication with patients is therapeutic and incorporates active listening are goals for the oncology nurse. Poor communication can cause significant suffering for both patients and families. The cancer experience, treatment side effects, and family dynamics can

---

Figure 6-4. Nutritional Guidelines for Patients With Ostomies

Hydration
Be sure to take adequate fluid to replace losses. The looser the stool, the more fluid that will be needed—at least 8–10 glasses per day.

Odor Control
Odor can be controlled with deodorants and filters.
Some foods that may cause odor include asparagus, eggs, cabbage, broccoli, cauliflower, garlic, onions, fish, and coffee. Parsley, cranberry juice, and yogurt may help to decrease odor.

Gas Control
Gas may be a problem for some people. It is important to try small amounts of foods of concern to determine if gas production will be a problem. Some foods that may produce gas include beer, broccoli, cabbage, cauliflower, brussels sprouts, cucumbers, beans, peas, peppers, and highly spiced foods. Avoiding gum chewing and drinking through straws may help to decrease gas, as can limiting pure sugars such as that found in gum, candy, and regular soft drinks.

Note. From "Colorectal Cancer" (p. 37), by K. Masino in V.J. Kogut and S.L. Luthringer (Eds.), *Nutritional Issues in Cancer Care*, 2005, Pittsburgh, PA: Oncology Nursing Society. Copyright 2005 by the Oncology Nursing Society. Reprinted with permission.

---

precipitate anxiety, depression, and maladaptive coping. The nurse can assess for psychosocial issues, teach about managing side effects, aid in decision making, and comfort patients and families. Communication skills are not innate, and many nurses have not evaluated their communication skills since college (Fallowfield et al., 2002). A recent review of the literature evaluated communication skills training programs for oncology healthcare professionals (Kennedy Sheldon, 2005). Communication skills, defined as specific behaviors and responses used in therapeutic relationships, were specifically taught in communication skills training programs. A variety of techniques and content was taught in these programs with desired outcomes of enhancing the repertoire of skills. Some improvement in communication skills and healthcare professional confidence in communicating with patients was noted, particularly in programs where training was reinforced. Significant gaps in the research literature, particularly for nurses, were noted (Kennedy Sheldon).

Review of the literature on communication needs of patients with cancer confirms these findings. Specific communication issues include the inability, either because of time restraints or lack of skill, of physicians to assess patients' information needs; physician domination of office visits, leaving patients with unmet communication needs; and differing recollections of communication about treatment options between physicians and patients (Hack, Degner, & Parker, 2005). Qualitative studies revealed that good communication, as perceived by patients, fostered feelings of control and mastery, and patient satisfaction scores were lowest concerning doctors' interpersonal skills and nurses' communication skills (Von Essen, Larsson, Oberg, & Sjoden, 2002). In one study of patients with metastatic disease, patients identified the following needs: communication within a caring relationship; open and repeated negotiations for patients' preferences; encouragement of hope and control; consistency of communication among members of the team; and attention to family members' needs, which may differ from those of the patient (Butow, Dowsett, Hagerty, & Tattersall, 2002).

Most of the literature on communication with patients and their families was conducted with breast cancer populations and needs to be expanded to other cancer types. Specific needs of people in minority groups, whether ethnic, socioeconomic, sexual orientation, or rural locale, need to be explored.

Quality of Life

Many disciplines have studied quality of life extensively, and the definition varies across specialties. This author prefers the definition of Ferrans and Powers (1992) of "a person's sense of well being that stems from satisfaction or dissatisfac-

tion with the areas of life that are important to him/her" (p. 29). The associated model (Ferrans, 1990) has been extensively researched and describes four major domains of quality of life: health and functioning, socioeconomic, psychological/spiritual, and family. As seen from this and other models, multiple factors can affect a patient's quality of life, highlighting the importance of comprehensive assessment and care planning (see Figure 6-5).

Providing compassionate care during suffering is an essential aspect of the oncology nurse's role. Patients who do not describe themselves as particularly spiritual still want care that gives them hope and provides meaning. The nurse can nurture the spirit of the patient in many ways, such as by being empathic and respectful, storytelling, encouraging self-expression (e.g., journal writing) and praying, and using humor (Taylor, 2003). Assisting a patient in finding meaning in his or her illness, such as changes in relationships, can be facilitated through acts of service or asking probing questions about the impact of the illness on his or her life and relationships.

Hope and its relationship to suffering have been described from numerous perspectives. From a nursing perspective, hope can be defined as a "multidimensional, dynamic life force characterized by a confident yet uncertain expectation of achieving a future good, which to the hoping person is

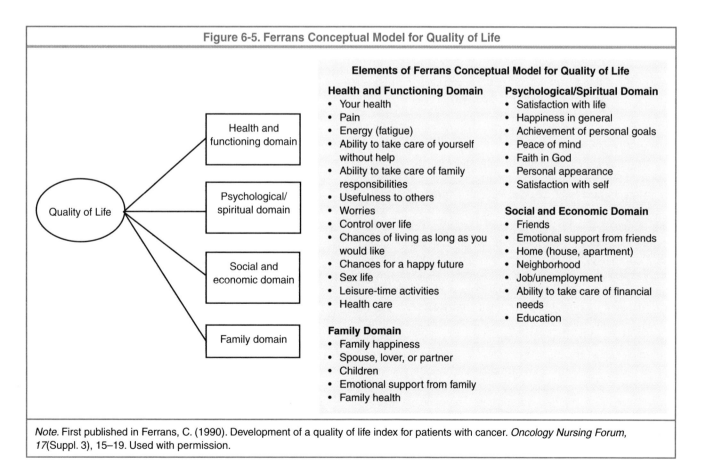

Figure 6-5. Ferrans Conceptual Model for Quality of Life

Elements of Ferrans Conceptual Model for Quality of Life

Health and Functioning Domain
- Your health
- Pain
- Energy (fatigue)
- Ability to take care of yourself without help
- Ability to take care of family responsibilities
- Usefulness to others
- Worries
- Control over life
- Chances of living as long as you would like
- Chances for a happy future
- Sex life
- Leisure-time activities
- Health care

Family Domain
- Family happiness
- Spouse, lover, or partner
- Children
- Emotional support from family
- Family health

Psychological/Spiritual Domain
- Satisfaction with life
- Happiness in general
- Achievement of personal goals
- Peace of mind
- Faith in God
- Personal appearance
- Satisfaction with self

Social and Economic Domain
- Friends
- Emotional support from friends
- Home (house, apartment)
- Neighborhood
- Job/unemployment
- Ability to take care of financial needs
- Education

Note. First published in Ferrans, C. (1990). Development of a quality of life index for patients with cancer. *Oncology Nursing Forum, 17*(Suppl. 3), 15–19. Used with permission.

realistically possible and personally significant" (Dufault & Martocchio, 1985, p. 380). Hope influences health and coping with illness. Ersek (2001) described cognitive strategies to maintain hope with life-threatening illness. These include appraising the illness as a challenge or test, reprioritizing one's life or engaging in service, joking about the illness, limiting the emotional response, relinquishing control to God, staying informed, fighting it or accepting the illness as God's will, living day to day, and identifying a history of personal strength. A substantial amount of excellent nursing research has been conducted in the area of maintaining or promoting hope in patients, and the reader is referred to the literature.

Nursing research has shed some light on patient coping after a CRC diagnosis. One study looked at couples adjusting to a diagnosis of colon cancer. In one case, the spouse reported significantly more emotional distress and less social support than the patient (Northouse, Mood, Templin, Mellon, & George, 2000). Women, in particular, reported more distress and less marital satisfaction, whether they were the patient or the spouse. Both patients and spouses reported decreases in their family functioning, but they also reported a decrease in emotional distress over time. Another study (Galloway & Graydon, 1996) found that patients discharged to home after CRC surgery had significant information needs about treatment, complications, and recovery. The more uncertain the patient felt, the more information needs he or she expressed. The authors concluded that increased attention to information needs at discharge may facilitate the patient's recovery at home.

The demands of illness and treatment of colon cancer greatly affect the functioning of patients and their families. Perception of these demands is derived from the person's view of the world, changes in role, decision-making processes, physical symptomatology, changes in self-image, uncertainty, and family relationship changes (Lewis, 1986; Woods, Yates, & Primomo, 1989). Klemm, Miller, and Fernsler (2000) examined the demands of illness in people (N = 121) treated for colorectal and anal cancers. Patients expressed illness-related concerns of an existential nature, and those patients with limited activity reported higher demands of illness. In another study examining the relationship between spiritual well-being and demands of illness in colorectal and anal cancers (Fernsler, Klemm, & Miller, 1999), people who reported higher levels of spiritual well-being expressed significantly lower demands of illness from symptoms and treatment. Men, younger people, those receiving treatment during the prior two months, and those with advanced disease and decreased activity reported the highest demands of illness. Based on this study, nurses should pay particular attention to younger patients, as their illness experience may be more difficult for them. The relationship between spiritual issues and the illness experience is an important one and attests to the need for nurses to engage in meaningful dialogue with patients about their spiritual needs.

Summary

This chapter has explored the broader issues involved in providing nursing care to people with GI cancers. Although significant advancements in treatment options have occurred over the past few years, the evidence behind much of nursing care is lacking. Preoperative and postoperative care, communication, anticipation of patients' informational needs, symptom management, and existential concerns are areas that should be explored.

References

American Society of Anesthesiologists Task Force on Preoperative Fasting. (1999). Practice guidelines for preoperative fasting and the use of pharmacologic agents to reduce the risk of pulmonary aspiration. *Anesthesiology, 90,* 896–905.

American Society for Gastrointestinal Endoscopy. (2001). *Colonoscopy preparations.* Retrieved April 9, 2006, from http://www.askasge.org/pages/tech/nt_colonoscopy.cfm

Bucher, P., Mermillod, B., Morel, P., & Soravia, C. (2004). Does mechanical bowel preparation have a role in preventing postoperative complications in elective colorectal surgery? *Swiss Medical Weekly, 134,* 69–74.

Butow, P., Dowsett, S., Hagerty, R., & Tattersall, M. (2002). Communication prognosis to patients with metastatic disease: What do they really want to know? *Supportive Care in Cancer, 10,* 161–168.

Colwell, J., & Fichera, A. (2005). Care of the obese patient with an ostomy. *Journal of Wound, Ostomy, and Continence Nursing, 32,* 378–383.

Crenshaw, J., & Winslow, E. (2002). Preoperative fasting: Old habits die hard: Research and published guidelines no longer support the routine use of "NPO after midnight," but the practice persists. *American Journal of Nursing, 102*(5), 36–44.

Dufault, K., & Martocchio, B. (1985). Hope: Its spheres and dimensions. *Nursing Clinics of North America, 20,* 379–391.

Enzinger, P.C., & Mayer, R.J. (2003). Esophageal cancer. *New England Journal of Medicine, 349,* 2241–2252.

Ersek, M. (2001). The meaning of hope in the dying. In B. Ferrell & N. Coyle (Eds.), *Textbook of palliative nursing* (pp. 339–351). New York: Oxford University Press.

Fallowfield, L., Jenkins, V., Farewell, V., Saul, J., Duffy, A., & Eves, R. (2002). Efficacy of a Cancer Research UK communication skills training model for oncologists: A randomised controlled trial. *Lancet, 359,* 650–656.

Fernsler, J., Klemm, P., & Miller, M. (1999). Spiritual well being and demands of illness in people with colorectal cancer. *Cancer Nursing, 22,* 134–140.

Ferrans, C. (1990). Quality of life: Conceptual issues. *Seminars in Oncology Nursing, 6,* 248–254.

Ferrans, C., & Powers, M. (1992). Psychometric assessment of the quality of life index. *Research in Nursing and Health, 15*(1), 29–38.

Galloway, S., & Graydon, J. (1996). Uncertainty, symptom distress and information needs after surgery for cancer of the colon. *Cancer Nursing, 19,* 112–117.

Gray, M., & Colwell, J. (2005). Mechanical bowel preparation before elective colorectal surgery. *Journal of Wound, Ostomy, and Continence Nursing, 32,* 360–364.

Grzelak, D. (2004). Management of patients with gastric and duodenal disorders. In S. Smeltzer & B. Bare (Eds.), *Brunner and*

Suddarth's textbook of medical surgical nursing (10th ed., pp. 1010–1027). Philadelphia: Lippincott Williams & Wilkins.

Guenaga, K., Matos, D., Castro, A., Atallah, A., & Wille-Jorgensen, P. (2005). Mechanical bowel preparation for elective colorectal surgery. *Cochrane Database for Systematic Reviews, 1.*

Hack, T., Degner, L., & Parker, P. (2005). The communication goals and needs of cancer patients: A review. *Psycho-Oncology, 14,* 831–845.

Itano, J. (2005). Cultural diversity among individuals with cancer. In C.H. Yarbro, M.H. Frogge, & M. Goodman (Eds.), *Cancer nursing: Principles and practice* (6th ed., pp. 70–94). Sudbury, MA: Jones and Bartlett.

Kennedy Sheldon, L. (2005). Communication in oncology care: The effectiveness of skills training workshops for healthcare providers. *Clinical Journal of Oncology Nursing, 9,* 305–312.

Klemm, P., Miller, M., & Fernsler, J. (2000). Demands of illness in people treated for colorectal cancer. *Oncology Nursing Forum, 27,* 633–639.

Lewis, F. (1986). The impact of cancer on the family: A critical analysis of the research literature. *Patient Education and Counseling, 8,* 269–289.

Madsen, D., Sebolt, T., Cullen, L., Folkedahl, B., Mueller, T., Richardson, C., et al. (2005). Listening to bowel sounds: An evidence-based practice project. *American Journal of Nursing, 105*(12), 40–50.

Manning, M. (2004). Management of patients with intestinal and rectal disorders. In S. Smeltzer & B. Bare (Eds.), *Brunner and Suddarth's textbook of medical-surgical nursing* (10th ed., pp. 1028–1073). Philadelphia: Lippincott Williams & Wilkins.

McCormick, D., Kibbe, P., & Morgan, S. (2002). Colon cancer: Prevention, diagnosis and treatment. *Gastroenterology Nursing, 25,* 204–211.

National Cancer Institute. (2004). *Photodynamic therapy for cancer: Questions and answers.* Retrieved April 9, 2006, from http://www.cancer.gov/cancertopics/factsheet/therapy/photodynamic

National Comprehensive Cancer Network. (2006a). *NCCN clinical practice guidelines in oncology: Colon/rectal cancer, version 2.2006.* Jenkintown, PA: Author.

National Comprehensive Cancer Network. (2006b). *NCCN clinical practice guidelines in oncology: Esophageal cancer, version 2.2006.* Jenkintown, PA: Author.

National Comprehensive Cancer Network. (2006c). *NCCN clinical practice guidelines oncology: Gastric cancer, version 2.2006.* Jenkintown, PA: Author.

National Institute of Diabetes and Digestive and Kidney Diseases. (2004). *National digestive diseases information clearinghouse.* Retrieved April 9, 2006, from http://digestive.niddk.nih.gov/

Northouse, L., Mood, D., Templin, T., Mellon, S., & George, T. (2000). Couples' pattern of adjustment to colon cancer. *Social Science and Medicine, 50,* 271–284.

O'Connor, K. (2005). Stomach cancer. In C.H. Yarbro, M.H. Frogge, & M. Goodman (Eds.), *Cancer nursing: Principles and practice* (6th ed., pp. 1617–1629). Sudbury, MA: Jones and Bartlett.

Perretta, S., Guerrero, V., & Garcia-Aguilar, J. (2006). Surgical treatment of rectal cancer. *Surgical Oncology Clinics of North America, 15*(1), 67–93.

Pisters, P., Kelsen, D., Powell, S., & Tepper, J. (2005). Cancer of the stomach. In V.T. DeVita, S. Hellman, & S. Rosenberg (Eds.), *Cancer: Principles and practice of oncology* (7th ed., pp. 909–944). Philadelphia: Lippincott Williams & Wilkins.

Posner, M.C., Forastiere, A.A., & Minsky, B. (2005). Cancer of the esophagus. In V.T. DeVita, S. Hellman, & S.A. Rosenberg (Eds.), *Cancer: Principles and practice of oncology* (pp. 861–908). Philadelphia: Lippincott Williams & Wilkins.

Ransohoff, D., & Sandler, R. (2002). Screening of colorectal cancer. *New England Journal of Medicine, 346,* 40–44.

Reilly, T., & Walker, G. (2004). Reasons for poor colonic preparation with inpatients. *Gastroenterology Nursing, 27,* 115–117.

Rossi, H., & Rothenberger, D. (2006). Surgical treatment of colon cancer. *Surgical Oncology Clinics of North America, 15*(1), 109–127.

Slim, K., Vicaut, E., Panis, Y., & Chipponi, J. (2004). Meta-analysis of clinical trials of colorectal surgery with or without mechanical bowel preparation. *British Journal of Surgery, 91,* 1125–1130.

Society of Gastroenterology Nurses and Associates. (1998). *Core curriculum for gastroenterology nursing* (2nd ed.). St. Louis, MO: Mosby.

Society of Gastroenterology Nurses and Associates. (2001). *Gastroenterology nursing: A core curriculum* (3rd ed.). Chicago: Author.

Society of Gastroenterology Nurses and Associates. (2003). *Manual of gastrointestinal procedures* (5th ed.). Chicago: Author.

Taylor, E. (2003). Spiritual quality of life. In C. King & P. Hinds (Eds.), *Quality of life: From nursing and patient perspectives* (2nd ed., pp. 93–116). Sudbury, MA: Jones and Bartlett.

Tsottles, N., & Reedy, A. (2005). Esophageal cancer. In C.H. Yarbro, M.H. Frogge, & M. Goodman (Eds.), *Cancer nursing: Principles and practice* (6th ed., pp. 1258–1274). Sudbury, MA: Jones and Bartlett.

Von Essen, L., Larsson, G., Oberg, K., & Sjoden, P. (2002). Satisfaction with care: Associations with health-related quality of life and psychosocial function among Swedish patients with endocrine gastrointestinal tumors. *European Journal of Cancer Care, 11,* 91–99.

Wilkes, G. (2005). Colon, rectal, and anal cancers. In C.H. Yarbro, M.H. Frogge, & M. Goodman (Eds.), *Cancer nursing: Principles and practice* (6th ed., pp. 1155–1214). Sudbury, MA: Jones and Bartlett.

Woods, N., Yates, B., & Primomo, J. (1989). Supporting families through chronic illness. *Image: The Journal of Nursing Scholarship, 21,* 46–50.

CHAPTER 7

Symptom Management of Gastrointestinal Cancers

Loleta Samuel-O'Garro, MSN, RN, APRN,BC, AOCN®, and
Sherri Henry Suozzo, MSN, APN-C, AOCN®

Introduction

This chapter focuses on symptom management for patients with gastrointestinal (GI) cancers. The symptoms discussed are selected based on prevalence in this population. The pathophysiology, etiology, symptoms, assessment, and interventions are described.

GI cancers usually are diagnosed in advanced stages of disease and often are preceded by nonspecific, ongoing symptoms, such as fatigue, malaise, anorexia, early satiety, postprandial fullness, weight loss, difficulty swallowing, changes in eating and bowel habits, and vague abdominal pain or cramping (Curtas, 1999; O'Connor, 1999).

Combined risk factors for GI cancers of the esophagus, stomach, liver, pancreas, colon, and rectum include tobacco use in conjunction with high alcohol consumption; diets high in nitrates (food such as pickled, fermented, cured, or processed meats) and low in vitamins A and C, protein, fruits, and vegetables; gastroesophageal reflux as seen with Barrett's esophagus; possible overexpression of the *p53* tumor suppressor gene; *Helicobacter (H.) pylori* infection; prior gastric resection; blood group A; pernicious anemia; achlorhydria; atrophic gastritis; family history; and obesity, ulcerative colitis, and Crohn disease (Glaser & Grogan, 1999; O'Connor, 1999; Quinn & Reedy, 1999; Saddler & Ellis, 1999).

Treatment of GI cancers involves the use of surgery, chemotherapy, and radiation therapy, often in combination but sometimes alone. Symptom management for patients with GI cancers is multidimensional and must be approached with the knowledge that most of the symptoms often are the result of multimodal therapy.

Chemotherapy is used in the neoadjuvant setting to decrease tumor size and facilitate surgical resection. In the adjuvant setting, it provides systemic therapy after surgery. Common chemotherapeutic agents used to treat GI cancers include, but are not limited to, cisplatin, 5-fluorouracil, bleomycin, mitomycin-C, doxorubicin, etoposide, metho-trexate, ifosfamide, streptozocin, gemcitabine, oxaliplatin, capecitabine, vinorelbine, and irinotecan.

Surgery often is used for curative resection or palliation. Radiation therapy is used for local control of tumor growth. Concurrent chemoradiation usually is reserved for patients for whom surgery is contraindicated because of advanced disease or inoperable tumors or in patients with multiple or nonstable comorbid conditions (Quinn & Reedy, 1999). In this setting, chemotherapy can enhance the effects of radiation therapy. Surgery may become an option after chemoradiation and may offer additional potential for cure.

Photodynamic therapy is less invasive than surgery and is used in the palliative care setting and for patients who are nonsurgical candidates. It involves the injection of a light-sensitive drug that migrates in high concentration to tumor cells. Then a fiberoptic probe with a light-bearing tip is used to activate the injected drug, and the tumor cells are killed.

Nutrition

Alterations in nutrition are common in patients with cancer. Nutritional status helps in the determination of the best treatment strategy; therefore, alterations in nutrition can lead to intolerance of treatment and complications of cancer therapy, such as secondary infections (Grant & Ropka, 1996). Nutritional alterations may be present before and after the cancer diagnosis and often are manifested in the subjective and objective experience of symptoms of anorexia, cachexia, weight loss, and malnutrition.

Weight Loss

The basic etiology of weight loss can be understood as the result of an increase in energy requirements and decreased intake. Weight loss in GI cancers primarily is related to mechanical disruptions in metabolism secondary to location of the tumor and from surgical intervention. Tumors may grow directly in locations along the GI tract and accessory organs and cause a mechanical interference with the normal transit of food. This may lead to inadequate intake or early satiety and poor absorption (Cunningham & Bell, 2000; O'Connor, 1999). Adjuvant or palliative surgical intervention disrupts the normal anatomy and may cause a deficiency of enzymes and hormones, as well as an inability to absorb some vitamins and minerals (e.g., B_{12}, iron) necessary for digestion and absorption (Cunningham & Bell; McGuire, 2000; O'Connor).

Dysphagia often contributes to weight loss secondarily as an adverse effect of mucositis from chemotherapy, tumor in the esophagus, or in relation to stenosis after esophagectomy. For stenosis, endoscopic dilation is indicated, with monitoring of the patient's neurologic status (gag reflex) afterward, then resumption of normal diet (McGuire, 2000; Quinn & Reedy, 1999).

Dumping Syndrome

Dumping syndrome is a postprandial event also known as vagotomy syndrome. Patients who have undergone surgery, such as esophagectomy and gastrectomy, are at the highest risk. The pathophysiology is not clear but may be related to the surgical interruption of the vagal nerve fibers that are important in conduction of impulses to the abdominal viscera. These fibers also play a role in the development of diarrhea. The anatomic changes from surgery may cause rapid emptying of hypertonic gastric contents (chyme) into the small bowel. The osmotic action of the food results in a rapid fluid shift into the lumen of the small intestine, which depletes the intravascular compartment and causes a release of peptide hormones and vasomotor symptoms. The patient experiences diarrhea, abdominal pain, dizziness, flushing, palpitation, nausea, vomiting, and fullness (McGuire, 2000; Quinn & Reedy, 1999). Patients also may experience gastroesophageal reflux because of the loss of the cardiac sphincter from the surgical procedure.

Onset of symptoms usually is within 20 minutes to two hours after a meal and may occur with each meal. Interventions for these patients are aimed at decreasing gastric emptying time and maximizing caloric intake. Patients should be instructed to eat small, frequent meals that contain fewer simple carbohydrates and increased protein and complex carbohydrates; limit fluids to between meals; avoid eating concentrated sugars; and sit up straight and avoid reclining for at least one hour after each meal. Taking pharmaceutical agents such as octreotide and loperamide before eating a meal also may be helpful (McGuire, 2000; Quinn & Reedy, 1999). Octreotide is a somatostatin analog that, when given before meals, may help patients with severe dumping syndrome because of its effects of binding to somatostatin receptors in the GI tract, suppressing GI contractions and thereby delaying or inhibiting GI transit time (Farooqi, Bevan, Sheppard, & Wass, 1999; Lamers, Bijlstra, & Harris, 1993). Loperamide is a peripherally acting opioid that slows GI transit time, en-

hances water and its absorption, and increases oral sphincter tone (Dunphy & Verne, 2001).

Anorexia-Cachexia Syndrome

Anorexia-cachexia syndrome is a multidimensional maladaptive response to physical and behavioral alterations in nutrition, which correlates with decreased quality of life and poor disease outcomes (Cunningham, 2004; Cunningham & Bell, 2000; Inui, 2002).

Anorexia can be defined as a loss of appetite or of compensatory increase in feeding that often leads to decreased food ingestion (Inui, 2002). Anorexia in patients with cancers of the GI tract may be related to pain, depression, malabsorption, constipation, mechanical obstructions, toxic or adverse effects to pain medications, or can occur with cancer treatment, such as chemotherapy or radiation therapy, which may cause changes in taste and smell (Inui, 2002).

Cachexia is profound involuntary weight loss and deterioration related to muscle wasting when protein and calorie requirements are not met (Cunningham & Bell, 2000). Conditions associated with cancer cachexia include those diagnosed with GI cancers, advanced cancers, use of nicotine-containing products, and preexisting digestive, metabolic, or absorptive disorders. Cachexia can occur as a primary or secondary response (Cunningham & Bell; Inui, 2002). The incidence of cancer cachexia is highest among patients with cancers of the stomach and pancreas; however, it also is associated with other cancers such as prostate, colon, and lung (McGuire, 2000). Its prevalence increases from 50%–80% before death and is the cause of mortality in more than 20% of patients with cancer (Inui, 2002).

Secondary cachexia occurs as a result of a functional inability to ingest or digest nutrients as a result of mechanical obstruction, malabsorption, or toxicity from treatment (Cunningham & Bell, 2000). Xerostomia, anorexia, nausea, vomiting, diarrhea, and dysgeusia/ageusia (altered or absent taste sensations) related to chemotherapy or radiation therapy can contribute to secondary cachexia. Surgical procedures that put patients at risk for dumping syndrome precipitate malabsorption (Cunningham & Bell).

Primary cachexia is characterized in the anorexia-cachexia syndrome, which develops as a result of a chronic systemic inflammatory response through progressive symptoms of anorexia, involuntary weight loss, and tissue wasting that eventually lead to poor performance status and sometimes death (Cunningham, 2004; Cunningham & Bell, 2000; Inui, 1999, 2002). When cachexia occurs, a loss of adipose tissue and skeletal muscle mass occurs, which is more pronounced with the progression of the disease as protein-calorie malnutrition advances (Inui, 1999, 2002).

Pathophysiologic mechanisms of the anorexia-cachexia syndrome demonstrate catabolic changes in metabolism of protein, fat, and carbohydrates mediated by lipid and protein mobilizing factors, cytokines, and some fatty acids (Cunningham & Bell, 2000; Inui, 2002). Protein loss occurs with reduced intake, reduced protein synthesis, and increased protein degradation. Decreased oral intake of carbohydrates threatens glucose availability for essential body processes by the brain and red blood cells (RBCs). Glucose stores in the liver and muscles are depleted, and protein eventually is degraded to become the primary source of energy. This leads to accelerated muscle wasting from protein loss. Loss of body fat occurs through decreased intake and increased fatty acid turnover (Cunningham, 2004; Inui, 2002).

Symptoms of anorexia-cachexia syndrome include decreased appetite, taste changes, early satiety, generalized weakness and fatigue, depletion of lean body mass, loss of body fat, changes in skin color and turgor, dehydration, hypotension, altered mobility, and mental status changes (Cunningham, 2004; Stepp & Pakiz, 2001).

Assessment of nutritional alterations should include a complete history and physical examination and an assessment of changes in appetite, food preferences, weight loss, height, weight, physical evidence of muscle wasting, and nutrient deficiencies. Laboratory evaluations should include a 24-hour urine collection for nitrogen balance; serum albumin and serum transferrin to check protein stores; RBC indices to assess iron stores; peripheral blood lymphocyte count to check for immunocompetence; plasma glucose to check for insulin resistance; and blood urea nitrogen and liver function tests (LFTs) to evaluate renal and hepatic function. A nutritional consultation should be arranged for assessment of dietary requirements (Cunningham, 2004).

Interventions for optimizing nutritional intake include pharmacologic appetite stimulants, oral nutritional supplements, enteral feedings, and total parenteral nutrition (Cunningham, 2004; Inui, 2002; McGuire, 2000).

Pharmacologic agents such as cannabinoids, antacids, prokinetic antiemetics, glucocorticoids, and synthetic progesterone are used in anorexia-cachexia syndrome and have demonstrated some improvement in nutritional intake through stimulation of appetite and decrease in nausea. They usually are given just before a meal, or they can be given at scheduled times around the clock (Inui, 2002; Sauter & Coleman, 1999). Glucocorticoids such as prednisolone, dexamethasone, and methylprednisolone have shown an average four-week limited effect of increased appetite and food intake, thus improving performance status and sense of well-being (Inui, 2002). Patients should be started on a one-week trial basis and given a bolus dose after breakfast or divided doses after breakfast and lunch to minimize steroid insomnia associated with late-day dosing. H_2 receptor antagonists should be used concurrently as prophylaxis against peptic ulceration (Inui, 2002).

Synthetic progesterones, such as megestrol acetate and medroxyprogesterone acetate, have demonstrated dose-related benefits of improved appetite and caloric intake and weight stabilization (Inui, 2002; Pascual Lopez et al., 2004).

Megestrol acetate is available as a pill or elixir and usually is started at doses of 160 mg/day with titration to an optimal dose of 800 mg/day with clinical response (Inui, 2002; Pascual Lopez et al.).

Metoclopramide is a prokinetic agent used for nausea but also has benefits of decreasing anorexia and early satiety. It is given in a slow-release form every 12 hours or as a 10 mg dose before each meal and at bedtime (Inui, 2002).

Cannabinoids such as marijuana and its derivatives (e.g., dronabinol [Marinol®, Solvay Pharmaceuticals, Marietta, GA]) are used for 24-hour appetite stimulation and should be given at bedtime to reduce euphoria, dizziness, confusion, and somnolence (Inui, 2002).

Postoperative Nutrition

Patients with GI cancers who have undergone surgical procedures may be started on liquid diets postoperatively and progress to semisolids and eventually solids by the time of discharge (Quinn & Reedy, 1999). Patients often are told to eat slowly, in smaller portions, and at more frequent intervals (i.e., eat six to eight small meals per day) (Quinn & Reedy). Following esophagectomy, patients should be instructed to eat any foods tolerated, as well as drink liquids between meals rather than with meals to help to prevent dumping syndrome (McGuire, 2000; Quinn & Reedy).

Changes in Taste and Smell

Patients may experience taste and smell alterations related to treatment. Recommendations should include using covered cookware in well-ventilated areas when preparing food and eating foods at room temperature, because they tend to have fewer odors and are better tolerated. Eating whole foods rather than processed foods and adding spices such as ginger and cinnamon may help to improve taste (Quinn & Reedy, 1999; Sauter & Coleman, 1999).

Enteral and Parenteral Nutrition

Parenteral nutrition is an ideal source of nutrition for patients who are unable to eat, digest, or absorb nutrients (McGuire, 2000). This route serves to improve energy stores and may decrease complications of treatment, resulting in an overall reduction of cost of care (McGuire; Sauter & Coleman, 1999).

A gastrostomy or jejunostomy tube may be placed for fluid balance and nutritional support after surgery or to manage side effects of treatment, such as dysphagia and mucositis (Quinn & Reedy, 1999). Tube feedings are started at a low rate, increased slowly, and discontinued once the patient's oral intake is adequate for nutritional needs (Quinn & Reedy).

For issues related to chemotherapy-induced nausea and vomiting, interventions should focus on comfort, adequate hydration, and optimal nutritional status. Recommendations should include eating lightly around treatment times and ingesting bland or creamy foods and snacks, such as ice, hard candy, and soda crackers. Patients should be encouraged to eat foods that are cold or room temperature and to decrease liquid intake with meals. Light exercise also may help to stimulate hunger (O'Connor, 1999; Sauter & Coleman, 1999).

Elimination

Third Spacing

Body fluids normally are contained in one of three compartmental spaces: intracellular, vascular, or interstitial. Fluid balance is managed at the level of the capillary membrane by the pull of opposing oncotic and osmotic pressures. Plasma proteins and other particulate matter also are exchanged at the capillary membrane level. Third spacing happens when a shift in fluid from the vascular to the interstitial spaces occurs as a result of low concentration of plasma proteins, changes in the opposing pressures at the capillary membrane, an increase in capillary permeability, lymphatic blockage, inflammation, or disease. Most commonly, generalized third spacing is seen in patients who are in septic shock or have undergone major surgical procedures such as pelvic exenteration or abdominoperineal resection.

There are two phases of third spacing—loss and reabsorption. In the loss phase, fluid shifts from the vascular to interstitial compartments. This usually happens immediately after surgery and can last for 48–72 hours. In the reabsorption phase, as the capillary pressures begin to normalize, interstitial fluid is reabsorbed into the vascular space. During this time, inflammation subsides, injured tissue heals, damaged capillaries are repaired, collateral lymphatics develop, and the degree of lymphatic blockage decreases (Miaskowski, 1996).

In the loss phase, the patient may appear hypovolemic and demonstrate hypotension, oliguria, low central venous pressure (CVP), increased urine-specific gravity, and tachycardia. Fluid intake may exceed output by a 3:1 ratio (Miaskowski, 1996). A marked increase in urine output is the hallmark of the reabsorption phase. Urine output may exceed 200 ml/hr (Miaskowski). Signs of hypervolemic shock, such as hypertension, weight gain, rales, dyspnea, elevated CVP, and jugular venous distention, may be present.

In the loss phase, treatment involves fluid and electrolyte replacement, plasma protein infusions, and use of diuretics. Infusion of plasma proteins such as albumin will help to rebalance the oncotic and osmotic pressures at the capillary membrane level and allow the fluid to shift from the interstitial back to the vascular compartments. Diuretics help to remove excess fluid that is reabsorbed and avoid vascular overload (Miaskowski, 1996). In the reabsorption phase, monitor the patient for signs of hypervolemia, and check fluid balance with intake and output. The amount of IV hydration supplied should be reduced.

Constipation

Patients with cancer of the GI tract often experience constipation; however, this symptom frequently is overlooked and undertreated. The pathophysiology of constipation in patients with GI cancer is complex and can vary greatly. Peristalsis moves stool through the bowel when increased stool volume causes stimulation. When stool is sensed in the rectum, the internal sphincter relaxes and allows passage of the stool through the external sphincter. Many factors affect the smooth muscles of the bowel, decreasing peristalsis and resulting in constipation (Cope, 2001). Consider three types of constipation when examining this patient population. Primary constipation is defined as being related to extrinsic factors such as diet and exercise. Secondary constipation encompasses bowel obstructions and metabolic effects, such as hypokalemia and excessive fluid loss secondary to vomiting. Iatrogenic constipation primarily is related to pharmacologic and medical interventions (Smith, 2001). Examples of causational factors include inadequate fluid intake, electrolyte imbalances, obstruction, neuropathy, opiate use, and anorectal disorders, such as an abscess or fissure (Nettina, 2001). Many patients with GI cancers have one or more of these factors, making constipation difficult to treat.

In addition to a complex pathophysiology, defining constipation is difficult. Every patient has different bowel habits; what one patient may consider constipation, another may consider normal. Therefore, evaluation of patients often is subjective. The first step in assessing constipation is obtaining a definition of what the patient considers constipation. This includes the size and consistency of the stool, frequency of bowel movements, and duration of the complaint (Arce, Ermocilla, & Costa, 2002). The Rome II Diagnostic Criteria for Functional Gastrointestinal Disorders is a tool that can be used for evaluating constipation. This tool defines functional constipation as straining, lumpy or hard stools, sensation of incomplete evacuation, sensation of anorectal blockage, and digital evacuation of more than one-quarter of stools passed and/or less than three defecations per week (Drossman, 2001). Using a standard tool to evaluate constipation may alleviate some of the ambiguity in treating and defining this symptom.

Little research looks at interventions used in alleviating constipation in patients with GI cancer; therefore, little evidence exists to guide decision making promoting evidence-based practice (Smith, 2001). Interventions include pharmacologic and nonpharmacologic measures or a combination of both. Initiating a bowel regimen often is beneficial in preventing constipation. This can be done by encouraging a regular pattern of defecation at the same time each day, increasing dietary fiber and fluid intake, and increasing physical activity for patients when appropriate (Wong & Kadakia, 1999).

Pharmacologic interventions for constipation include four groups of laxatives that act in different ways: bulk-forming, stool softeners, stimulants, and osmotic laxatives. Generally, the first line of treatment for cancer-related constipation is bulk-forming laxatives, such as psyllium or methylcellulose. When a patient is on a bulk-forming laxative, he or she must have an adequate intake of fluids for the laxative to work, which may be difficult for older adults or patients with a poor performance status. Also, bulk-forming laxatives are not appropriate for opioid-induced constipation (McMillan, 2002; Smith, 2001). Side effects associated with bulk-forming laxatives include abdominal cramping and bloating. These adverse effects can be alleviated by gradually increasing the dose of bulk-forming laxative (Avila, 2004).

Second-line pharmacologic interventions for primary constipation include incorporating an emollient stool softener such as docusate sodium with a stimulant such as senna into the bowel regimen. These laxatives are combined because emollient laxatives serve little value alone in the treatment of constipation but work well in combination with stimulants and bulk-forming laxatives by softening the stool (Avila, 2004). If constipation persists after initiation of an emollient and stimulant, an osmotic laxative, such as lactulose, may be introduced. Table 7-1 lists the advantages and disadvantages of each class of laxatives, with the suggested role of each in therapy.

Secondary constipation caused by pathologic changes may not be amenable to prevention. In these cases, medical interventions, such as surgery or electrolyte repletion, may be necessary. Secondary constipation may be severe and even life threatening and always should be considered in a patient with GI cancer (McMillan, 2002).

Table 7-1. Pharmacologic Treatment of Constipation

Type of Laxative	Advantages	Disadvantages	Suggested Role in Therapy
Bulk-forming Methylcellulose Psyllium Polycarbophil	Most closely mimics the physiologic mechanism in promoting evacuation; useful in patients with colostomies	May take up to three days for effect; increased gas and bloating during initiation of therapy; potential for drug-drug interaction when administered with other medications; significant hydration required; contraindicated in patients who have obstructive symptoms or fecal impaction	Ideal as a first-line agent in cases of mild or transient constipation not associated with opioid-induced constipation
Emollient Docusate	Effective stool softener, particularly in cases where painful defecation and straining need to be avoided; available in tablets or liquid formulations	Increased fluid intake required; increased risk of absorption of poorly absorbed drugs when given concurrently; unpleasant taste of liquid formulation	First-line agent administered concomitantly with stimulant laxatives in the prevention of iatrogenic constipation; beneficial when given with bulk-forming agents to reduce straining
Lubricant Mineral oil	Useful in situations of excessive straining	Chronic use may lead to malabsorption of fat-soluble vitamins; risk of possible aspiration when given orally; enhanced toxicity when given with docusate	Not routinely recommended
Osmotic Lactulose Sorbitol Glycerin PEG with electrolytes PEG without electrolytes	Useful in liquefying stools to allow for defecation; sorbitol less nauseating than lactulose	May cause abdominal pain and distention shortly after ingestion; excessive bloating and colic with larger doses of lactulose; sweet taste may exacerbate underlying nausea.	Second-line therapy when a stimulant laxative and stool softener do not relieve constipation
Stimulant Bisacodyl Senna Cascara Castor oil (ricinoleic acid) Casanthranol (with docusate)	Useful in liquefying stools to allow for defecation	Long-term use associated with development of melanosis coli, cathartic colon, and potentially cancer; discoloration of urine; may need to titrate to higher doses (multiple daily tablets for adequate control; may cause abdominal cramping and hypokalemia)	First-line (senna) for prevention of opioid-induced constipation; may be used as first-line therapy in combinations with stool softener; useful in iatrogenic constipation (vincas, 5HT$_3$ antagonists)

Note. From "Pharmacologic Treatment of Constipation in Cancer Patients," by J.G. Avila, 2004, *Cancer Control, 11*(Suppl. 3), pp. 11–18. Copyright 2004 by Moffitt Cancer Center. Adapted with permission.

Diarrhea

Normally, the GI tract functions to absorb and digest nutrients. Diarrhea frequently is seen in patients with GI cancers and is both a sign and a symptom. The definition of diarrhea is an abnormal increase in stool liquidity and frequency. Diarrhea can be acute or chronic and can be associated with other symptoms such as abdominal cramping, incontinence, and the urge to defecate. Diarrhea can be a result of treatment or the disease process. If left untreated, diarrhea can cause serious complications, contributing to morbidity and mortality, and must be managed effectively (Engelking, 2003).

Pathophysiology of diarrhea in the patient with GI cancer also is complex. Several types of diarrhea may occur in this patient population, including osmotic, malabsorptive, secretory, exudative, dysmotility associated, and chemotherapy induced (Engelking, 2003). Osmotic diarrhea is characterized by a large volume of watery stools, which is caused by a mechanical disturbance due to an influx of fluid and electrolytes into the intestinal lumen. This fluid overwhelms the bowel and affects the absorption of fluids. Osmotic diarrhea can be caused by ingestion of hyperosmolar substances, such as enteral tube feedings (Rutledge & Engelking, 1998). Malabsorptive diarrhea results when a disturbance occurs in both mechanical and biochemical functions responsible for mediating the absorptive process. A large volume of foul-smelling stool is indicative of this. Diarrhea associated with colon surgery is an example of malabsorptive diarrhea. Because of the decrease in the surface area of the colon, a decrease occurs in the absorptive ability of the colon. This causes an increase of osmotically active substances entering the colon, which stimulates the bowel (Rutledge & Engelking). Secretory diarrhea occurs when there is an increase in production of potent endogenous diarrheogenic substances. Endocrine tumors, bacteria, gut wall damage as seen in graft-versus-host disease, and short gut syndrome can produce these substances. Secretory diarrhea manifests itself with a large volume of watery stools that persists even after fasting (Engelking; Rutledge & Engelking). Exudative diarrhea is caused by a discharge of mucus, serum protein, or blood into the bowel, causing inflammation. It is commonly referred to as inflammatory diarrhea. Exudative diarrhea is characterized by a variable volume but a high frequency of stools. This type of diarrhea is seen in patients receiving pelvic radiation. Dysmotility-associated diarrhea occurs when intestinal motility becomes erratic in response to alterations in the stretch receptors of the bowel that determine peristaltic activity. Frequent, small, semisolid stools are noted in this type of diarrhea. Dysmotility-associated diarrhea is seen in patients with fecal impactions and with opiate use (Engelking; Rutledge & Engelking). The pathophysiology of chemotherapy-induced diarrhea is complex. Sloughing of the epithelial mucosa without replacement of the basement membrane, a toxicity of some chemotherapeutic agents, causes superficial ulceration and extensive bowel wall inflammation.

Frequent watery to semisolid stools occur 24–96 hours after treatment. Figure 7-1 lists chemotherapeutic agents that are associated with chemotherapy-induced diarrhea.

Figure 7-1. Common Chemotherapeutic Agents Associated With Diarrhea

- Irinotecan
- Cisplatin
- Fluorouracil
- Oxaliplatin
- Docetaxel
- Capecitabine

Assessment of diarrhea begins with a diarrhea-focused history. A focused history is a valuable tool and an important intervention that the oncology nurse can implement autonomously. A focused history should include details about the onset, duration, frequency, timing, volume, appearance, and aggravating and alleviating factors of the diarrhea. Additional information includes fluid intake and change in weight (Viele, 2003). The National Cancer Institute Common Terminology Criteria for Adverse Events (CTCAE) also is a useful tool in assessing diarrhea (see Table 7-2). These criteria can be found online at http://ctep.cancer.gov/reporting/ctc.html. The nurse cannot begin to incorporate interventions until the history is evaluated.

Nutritional interventions should be initiated once the focused history has been evaluated. Encourage the patient to eat small, frequent meals, minimize fluid intake with meals, and eat foods that are high in electrolytes, such as potassium. It is also important to teach the patient what foods to avoid. Foods associated with increasing diarrhea include spices such as curry or cayenne pepper, high-fat foods, alcohol, caffeine, dairy products, and juices high in sorbitol, such as prune juice (Stern & Ippoliti, 2003).

Pharmacologic management is an important intervention in managing diarrhea. Categories of antidiarrheal medications include intestinal transit inhibitors that prolong transit time through the bowel and antisecretory agents that decrease fluid secretion. The most commonly prescribed medications for first-line treatment of diarrhea in patients with cancer include intestinal transit inhibitors such as loperamide and diphenoxylate plus atropine. Loperamide is initiated at 4 mg every two to four hours up to 16 mg/day (Stern & Ippoliti, 2003). Loperamide is especially useful in the treatment of irinotecan-induced diarrhea. Adverse effects of loperamide generally are mild, and the drug is well tolerated. Diphenoxylate plus atropine often is used as first-line treatment of cancer treatment–induced diarrhea. It is administered as a tablet in doses of diphenoxylate 2.5 mg/atropine 0.025 mg up to a maximum of eight tablets per day. Adverse reactions are more common than with loperamide and include flushing, tachycardia, dry

Table 7-2. Common Terminology Criteria for Adverse Events: Diarrhea

Adverse Event	Grade				
	1	2	3	4	5
Diarrhea*	Increase of < 4 stools per day over baseline; mild increase in ostomy output compared to baseline	Increase of 4–6 stools per day over baseline; IV fluids indicated < 24 hours; moderate increase in ostomy output compared to baseline; not interfering with activities of daily living	Increase of ≥ 7 stools per day over baseline; incontinence; IV fluids ≥ 24 hours; hospitalization; severe increase in ostomy output compared to baseline; interfering with activities of daily living	Life-threatening consequences (e.g., hemodynamic collapse)	Death

*Diarrhea includes diarrhea of small bowel or colonic origin and/or ostomy diarrhea.

Note. Based on information from the National Cancer Institute Cancer Therapy Evaluation Program, 2003.

mouth, urinary retention, and sedation. This drug should not be used in patients with renal or liver impairment (Stern & Ippoliti). Atropine also can be used alone in the treatment of acute onset diarrhea during treatment with irinotecan. This acute diarrhea is described as cramping diarrhea occurring within 24 hours of the irinotecan infusion. A dose of atropine at 0.25 mg can be administered intravenously or subcutaneously prior to irinotecan or when symptoms appear (Stern & Ippoliti). A life-threatening GI syndrome can be seen in patients receiving the combination therapy of irinotecan, fluorouracil, and leucovorin. This syndrome presents as acute diarrhea, nausea, vomiting, anorexia, and abdominal cramping. Symptoms are associated with severe dehydration, neutropenia, fever, and electrolyte imbalances (Rothenberg, Meropol, Poplin, Van Cutsem, & Wadler, 2001). Aggressive management of diarrhea associated with this treatment regimen is recommended, including the use of loperamide and an oral fluoroquinolone at the initiation of therapy. If delayed diarrhea occurs, patients are instructed to take loperamide 2 mg orally every 2 hours during the day and 4 mg orally every 4 hours at night until they are diarrhea-free for 12 hours. If diarrhea persists more than 24 hours, patients are to begin the fluoroquinolone and take the medication for seven days. If diarrhea persists more than 48 hours, patients are hospitalized (Rothenberg et al.). The oncology nurse can play an important role during this time by reinforcing the teaching during treatment and evaluating the incidence of diarrhea during office visits and through telephone contact.

Patients who do not respond to intestinal transit inhibitors may be treated with octreotide, an antisecretory medication. Octreotide is administered three times a day subcutaneously at a dose of 500 micrograms. Octreotide also is useful in the treatment of radiation-induced diarrhea (Stern & Ippoliti, 2003). The STOP (Sandostatin LAR Depot Trial for the Optimum Prevention of Chemotherapy-Induced Diarrhea) trial currently is evaluating two different dose levels (30 mg

and 40 mg) of octreotide LAR in reducing the incidence of chemotherapy-induced diarrhea (Anthony, 2003). Hopefully answers will be available soon about the dosing, efficacy, and tolerability of this drug.

Mucous Membranes

Mucositis

The alimentary tract is lined with soft, smooth layers of epithelial cells and connective tissue that are self-renewing. The basement epithelial cells are replaced about every 3–5 days with a resultant turnover rate of the outer lining every 7–14 days (Grant & Kravits, 2000; Sonis, 2004). The purpose of this lining is protection, absorption of nutrients and water, and secretion of enzymes, mucus, and salts (Grant & Kravits). The use of irritants, such as tobacco and alcohol, or damage of this lining, such as with chemotherapy or radiation therapy, results in inflammation of the mucous membranes, or mucositis (Grant & Kravits; Quinn & Reedy, 1999). Untreated mucositis may lead to secondary associated symptoms such as local or systemic infection, anorexia, dehydration, weight loss from poor oral intake, and deficiencies in proteins and vitamins (Avritscher, Cooksley, & Elting, 2004; Brown & Wingard, 2004; Grant & Kravits; Sonis).

Mucositis can occur in the oral cavity as stomatitis (inflammation of the oropharyngeal mucosa) or in the GI tract as esophagitis (inflammation of the esophageal mucosa), enteritis (inflammation of the intestinal mucosa), and proctitis (inflammation of the anorectal mucosa). Pain is a common symptom with mucositis and is secondary to the cell injury/damage that stimulates the inflammatory response, during which there is a release of neurotransmitters and stimulation of nociceptive pain fibers in the mucosa (Grant & Kravits, 2000; Peterson, Beck, & Keefe, 2004).

Risk factors for the development of mucositis and the duration of symptoms can be patient and/or treatment related. Patient-related factors include age, gender, oral hygiene practices, tobacco and alcohol use, previous cancer therapy, and nutritional status, especially protein malnutrition. Treatment-related factors include chemotherapy dose, regimen, and schedule, with or without concomitant radiation therapy (Avritscher et al., 2004; Brown & Wingard, 2004; Grant & Kravits, 2000).

Women tend to have a greater risk than men for mucositis with fluorouracil-based chemotherapy (Avritscher et al., 2004). The impact of age is not fully understood, but children and older adults are at greatest risk. Children may be at greater risk for severe stomatitis and enteritis related to a higher proliferation rate of mucosal cells and a high degree of immunosuppression during cancer therapy (Avritscher et al.). Older adults may be affected because of reduced renal function that may increase toxicity of the chemotherapeutic agents. The decrease in renal function plus an age-related decline in stem cell reserve compromises tissue loss recovery (Avritscher et al.).

Poor oral hygiene practices resulting in dental caries and gum disease predispose patients to a higher risk for stomatitis and oral infection during cancer therapy. Xerostomia, or dry mouth, related to a decreased flow of saliva from some medications (antidepressants), radiation therapy to the head and neck, and chemotherapy decrease the bactericidal proteins that normally wash the mucosal lining of the oral cavity and also can contribute to stomatitis (Avritscher et al., 2004).

Myelosuppression with a decreased neutrophil count during chemotherapy offers an opportunistic period for overgrowth of the endogenous flora (gram-positive and gram-negative bacteria, fungi, and viruses) of the alimentary mucosa, which may lead to local or systemic infections (Grant & Kravits, 2000). Chemotherapeutic agents such as fluorouracil, vinorelbine, mitomycin-C, bleomycin, doxorubicin, irinotecan, methotrexate, and etoposide used to treat GI cancers potentiate the risk for mucositis (Avritscher et al., 2004; Brown & Wingard, 2004; Grant & Kravits). Etoposide and methotrexate are secreted in saliva and therefore have direct, marked oral mucotoxicity (Avritscher et al.). Irinotecan is associated with severe enteritis, usually demonstrated as secretory, delayed diarrhea (Avritscher et al.). The severity of mucositis is related to the dose and schedule of the chemotherapy. Oral mucositis is twice as common as GI mucositis, usually with an onset of five to seven days after the start of chemotherapy and a peak at day 14 (Avritscher et al.; Grant & Kravits; Keefe, Gibson, & Hauer-Jensen, 2004). Symptoms of GI mucositis usually peak within three days of chemotherapy (Keefe et al.). Overall, mucositis often resolves within two to three weeks (Avritscher et al.; Grant & Kravits; Keefe et al.).

Radiation therapy to the GI tract may cause cell damage, collagen destruction, and atrophy of the lining. Mucosal thinning can become a long-term mucotoxic effect from radiation therapy and may lead to chronic, nonhealing ulceration that could progress to tissue necrosis, obstruction, strictures, and perforation (Avritscher et al., 2004; Keefe et al., 2004).

Primary symptoms in oral mucositis include erythema, oral ulcers/lesions, dysgeusia/ageusia (altered or absent taste sensations), pain, difficulty eating, and xerostomia (Brown & Wingard, 2004; Sonis, 2004). Good oral hygiene is recommended for both prevention and treatment of oral mucositis. Preventive measures for oral mucositis focus on maintaining tissue stability and reducing tissue irritation and oral microbial colonization (Epstein & Schubert, 2004). Specific recommendations include regular brushing and flossing of the teeth, adequate fluid intake to improve salivation, and decreased or eliminated consumption of alcohol and highly acidic or spicy foods. During chemotherapy or radiation therapy, oral hygiene should be performed every four hours while awake. Patients should be encouraged to eat food high in protein and calories and to increase the intake of vitamins B and C.

Cryotherapy with ice is used during the infusion of some chemotherapeutic agents, such as fluorouracil, to reduce the degree of mucositis. Ice promotes local vasoconstriction, thereby decreasing the circulation of the agent (i.e., fluorouracil) to the oral mucosa during peak blood levels. Decreasing the circulating drug during peak levels protects the layers of proliferating epithelial cells and decreases local cytotoxicity. This form of cryotherapy entails the use of ice chips in the oral cavity for 5 minutes before and 25 minutes after fluorouracil bolus administration (Koppel & Boh, 2001; Peterson et al., 2004). Cryotherapy is not recommended for continuous infusion of fluorouracil (Peterson et al.).

Symptoms of esophagitis include substernal chest pain, dysphagia (difficulty swallowing), odynophagia (pain on swallowing), difficulty talking, and dyspepsia (Keefe et al., 2004). Treatment involves the use of local anesthetics, analgesics, H_2 blockers or proton pump inhibitors, spasmolytics, possible interruption of radiation therapy, and esophageal dilation if strictures occur (Keefe et al.).

Enteritis may involve the stomach, small intestine, and colon. The patient may exhibit symptoms of gastritis, nausea, bloating, diarrhea, and abdominal pain. In the case of radiation-induced enteritis, acute nausea may occur early during the treatment, whereas abdominal pain and diarrhea occur two to three weeks into treatment. These symptoms usually resolve within two to four weeks after completion of therapy (Keefe et al., 2004). In patients with chronic radiation toxicity, latent symptoms may occur as intermittent constipation, malnourishment, dysmetabolism, fibrotic strictures, localized ischemia, perforation, or formation of fistulas (Keefe et al.). Treatment for acute enteritis includes the use of antidiarrheal medications and antiemetics (Keefe et al.).

Pharmacologic interventions for mucositis are topical agents, systemic analgesics, and antimucotoxic agents. Pharmacotherapy with topical agents includes the use of local anesthetics, analgesics, and coating agents. Patients should be instructed on proper use and results of the various agents. Viscous lidocaine is a topical anesthetic used for patients with oral mucositis to help with pain relief. It has limited systemic absorption, can anesthetize taste, and may sting with initial application; the effects usually last for 15–30 minutes. Patients should be monitored for suppression of the gag reflex because of anesthesia of the oropharynx (Epstein & Schubert, 2004). Benzydamine is a nonsteroidal, anti-inflammatory analgesic and mucoprotective oral rinse. When used prophylactically, benzydamine may help to reduce the incidence and severity of treatment-induced mucositis (Epstein & Schubert; Peterson et al., 2004). Gelclair® (OSI Pharmaceuticals, Inc., Melville, NY) is an oral gel analgesic that forms an adherent barrier to protect the oral mucosa (Epstein & Schubert). Gelclair is available only by prescription. Doxepin, a tricyclic antidepressant, has been used effectively as a topical analgesic (Epstein & Schubert). Doxepin rinse 5 mg/ml plus 0.1% alcohol plus sorbitol has demonstrated analgesic efficacy for oral mucosal pain due to cancer therapy (Epstein et al., 2001).

Sucralfate and liquid antacids have been used as coating agents for stomatitis and enteritis. Liquid antacids are used in "magic mouthwash" combinations that include a topical anesthetic and antihistamine. Sucralfate has demonstrated benefits when used as an enema in radiation proctitis at a dose of 2 g in 20 ml water per rectum twice daily (Grant, 1999).

H_2 blockers, such as ranitidine, or proton pump inhibitors, such as omeprazole, also are used prophylactically to reduce chemotherapy-induced esophagitis (Keefe et al., 2004).

Skin

Hand-Foot Syndrome

Hand-foot syndrome (HFS) is a localized, cutaneous, drug-specific, dose-limiting toxicity of chemotherapy also known as acral erythema or palmar-plantar erythrodysesthesia. It is commonly related to continuous infusion of fluorouracil and doxorubicin but also can be seen with the use of capecitabine and liposomal doxorubicin (Childress & Lokich, 2003; Gerbrecht, 2003; Koppel & Boh, 2001; Scheithauer & Blum, 2004). Although HFS is not life threatening, it can be debilitating and interferes with quality of life.

The actual pathophysiology of HFS is not clear. The syndrome is most likely not related to the catabolism of doxorubicin or fluorouracil because these drugs are of two different classes, yet they produce the exact symptoms of HFS with both continuous or protracted infusions of each (Childress & Lokich, 2003; Gerbrecht, 2003; Quinn & Reedy, 1999).

Clinical symptoms occur in as many as 25% of patients receiving continuous or protracted infusions of fluorouracil and doxorubicin (Childress & Lokich, 2003) and 50% of patients receiving capecitabine therapy (Piguet & Borradori, 2002). The symptoms of HFS may evolve rapidly in three grades. Patients with grade 1 symptoms demonstrate a prodromal period of tingling or pain followed by intense, painful, confluent, well-defined erythema of the palmar and plantar surfaces. If the drug infusion continues, grade 2 symptoms develop with continued tingling and dysesthesia along with progressive swelling of these surfaces and, eventually, the formation of giant bullae, particularly along pressure surfaces of the heels and metatarsals (Childress & Lokich; Gerbrecht, 2003). Grade 3 symptoms are characterized by blistering and desquamation of the affected surfaces (Childress & Lokich; Gerbrecht).

Interventions for HFS are aimed at ameliorating symptoms, but insufficient clinical evidence is available to support their use (Scheithauer & Blum, 2004). Treatment modification with interruption or dose reduction of chemotherapy often will halt progression and is the only proven strategy (Scheithauer & Blum). Symptomatic and prophylactic treatments include the use of creams and lotions, cooling of the affected areas, and pharmacotherapy.

Topical ammonium lactate lotion (Lac-Hydrin®, Bristol-Myers Squibb, Princeton, NJ), hemp-based creams (Aquaphor®, Smith & Nephew, Andover, MA), lanolin creams, and Bag Balm® (Vermont's Original, Lyndonville, VT) are examples of soothing emollients used to relieve the surface discomfort of HFS and can be started before or with the appearance of symptoms. These topical agents should be applied regularly, with particular attention to skin creases on the palmar and plantar surfaces. Pyridoxine 50–150 mg three times a day can be prescribed concurrently with infusion of the chemotherapy, or it may be administered when symptoms occur to relieve dysesthesia. Cool compresses applied to the affected extremities during chemotherapy infusion may help to alleviate symptoms to allow continuance of treatment. Soft pads or socks worn inside shoes and cotton gloves will help to cushion sore skin (Childress & Lokich, 2003; Gerbrecht, 2003; Koppel & Boh, 2001; Nagore, Insa, & Sanmartin, 2000).

A second form of HFS related to the use of docetaxel has been observed. A suggested name for it is periarticular thenar erythema and oncolysis (PATEO), and it occurs in less than 5% of patients. PATEO is more common with weekly treatment versus an every-three-week schedule. Clinical symptoms appear as reddish purple discolorations of the skin on the Achilles tendon and dorsal surfaces of the hands, particularly at the base of the thumb or hypothenar areas. Erythema may progress to blistering and desquamation. Nail bed changes may progress to oncolysis (Childress & Lokich, 2003).

Pruritus

The term *pruritus* often is used interchangeably with itching. It is a localized or generalized unpleasant sensation in the superficial layers of skin, conjunctivae, mucous membranes, and upper respiratory tract that provokes a desire to scratch (Etter & Myers, 2002; Lidstone & Thorns, 2001; Yarbro & Seiz, 2004). Scratching may damage skin integrity and lead to excoriation and erythema. This threatens the skin's role as a barrier organ and may promote infection. Pruritus can lead to changes in quality of life because of severe discomfort, sleep disturbances, social embarrassment, and difficulty in concentrating (Davis, Frandsen, Walsh, Andresen, & Taylor, 2003; Etter & Myers; Lidstone & Thorns; Yarbro & Seiz).

The pathophysiology of pruritus is not fully understood. A balanced network of blood vessels, mast cells, and connective nerve fibers exists in the layers of skin. Within this network, there are many central and peripheral mediators of pruritus. These include histamine; serotonin; neuropeptides such as substance P, calcitonin, and vasoactive intestinal peptide; endogenous opioids; proteases; cytokines; and growth factors and eicosanoids, such as prostaglandins E2, H_2, and leukotrienes (Davis et al., 2003; Etter & Myers, 2002; Lidstone & Thorns, 2001; Twycross et al., 2003; Yarbro & Seiz, 2004).

Stimulation of the cutaneous nerve endings located at the junction of the epidermis and dermis sends impulses along pathways of unmyelinated nerve fibers (similar to the pain-conducting fibers) to the dorsal root ganglia, continuing to the thalamus, and then to the somatosensory cortex in the brain. This results in a sensory perception of an itch, followed by a motor response of an urge to scratch. This becomes a cycle that may result in tissue destruction because the urge to scratch often is irresistible; and although scratching produces a pleasurable relief from the itch, it causes a release of the main peripheral chemical mediator histamine by the mast cells present in layers of the skin and circulates basophils. When histamine is released, the sensation of itching is increased (Etter & Myers, 2002; Lidstone & Thorns, 2001; Twycross et al., 2003; Yarbro & Seiz, 2004).

Pruritus may be localized or generalized. Localized pruritus may be triggered by dry skin and irritation from dermatologic conditions or radiation therapy. Generalized pruritus may be associated with malignancies, cholestasis, uremia/renal failure, opioid use, drug reactions, chemotherapy use, or metabolic problems (Etter & Myers, 2002; Gallagher, 1995). Malignancies associated with pruritus include lymphomas, myeloma, glioblastoma, melanoma, and cancer of the vulva. Paraneoplastic syndromes from cancers of the cervix, prostate, colon, rectum, anus, stomach, and others also are associated with pruritus (Lidstone & Thorns, 2001).

Assessment of pruritus involves a complete history for symptom onset, duration, location, aggravating and relieving factors, current medications, and past medical history. Examination should include observation and documentation of skin condition/lesions, biopsy of suspicious skin lesions, and laboratory testing that includes erythrocyte sedimentation rate, LFTs, and renal function tests (Lidstone & Thorns, 2001).

Management of pruritus can be divided into general and pharmaceutical measures. General measures are aimed at prevention of dry skin and irritation, whereas pharmaceutical agents may help to treat all or specific causes of pruritus.

General interventions for pruritus should include recommendations for activities that would minimize exacerbation of pruritus, such as avoid alcohol and spicy foods, wear lightweight clothing, maintain a cool environment, keep nails short, and gently rub the skin rather than scratch it (Lidstone & Thorns, 2001). Further recommendations include measures for soothing and hydrating skin through the use of tepid, lukewarm water and mild soaps or oatmeal additives for baths, rinsing the skin well, and limiting baths to 10–20 minutes per day. Hot baths are not encouraged because heat causes vasodilation of blood vessels and can increase itching. After bathing, patients should regularly use moisturizing agents, such as bath oils or emollient lubricants, and avoid perfumes and starch-based powders on the skin. Baking soda is preferable to deodorants to avoid axillary irritation (Gallagher, 1995; Lidstone & Thorns; Twycross et al., 2003; Yarbro & Seiz, 2004). For pruritus associated with jaundice, interventions include using sodium bicarbonate baths, applying topical lotions with calamine and cocoa butter, and using detergents and soaps sparingly (Sauter & Coleman, 1999).

Pharmacotherapy for pruritus includes the use of topical and systemic agents in a localized or generalized setting. Topical preparations for localized pruritus include over-the-counter preparations with corticosteroids, astringents, antihistamines, or moisturizers. Corticosteroid creams are useful for pruritus associated with localized inflammation. Menthol or phenol in aqueous creams is useful for soothing irritation. Capsaicin cream depletes substance P from the nerve fibers and is helpful in decreasing pain and itching. Capsaicin may cause a burning sensation on initial application, making it poorly tolerated and decreasing compliance and generalized application (Lidstone & Thorns, 2001; Twycross et al., 2003). Phenol containing calamine lotion sometimes is used as an astringent; however, its drying effect is counterproductive, so use should be limited to pruritic, weeping, and vesicular lesions (Twycross et al.; Yarbro & Seiz, 2004).

Multiple classes of systemic agents are useful in treating pruritus. H_1 receptor antagonist antihistamines, such as chlorphenamine and cetirizine, are useful in pruritus mediated primarily by histamines, such as with insect bites, urticaria, and drug rashes. H_2 receptor antagonists, such as cimetidine, also are helpful with pruritus for hematologic conditions because they enhance the effects of H_1 receptor antagonists and inhibit hepatic cytochrome CYP2D6 (Twycross et al., 2003). Opioid antagonists, such as parenteral naloxone or oral naltrexone, help with pruritus from cholestasis or opioid use. $5HT_3$ receptor blockers, such as ondansetron, relieve pruritus from spinal opioid use, cholestasis, and renal failure. Selective serotonin reuptake inhibitors, such as paroxetine, help with pruritus associated with cholestasis, opioid use, and paraneoplastic disorders (Etter & Myers, 2002; Lidstone & Thorns, 2001; Twycross et al.; Zylicz, Krajnik, Sorge, & Costantini, 2003). Tricyclic antidepressants, such as doxepin and amitriptyline, have potent H_1- and/or H_2-receptor blocker activity useful in combating pruritus but should be discontinued at least two weeks before starting a monoamine oxidase inhibitor. Doxepin is available for use as a topical cream (avoid use in children) or in pill form and should not be used concurrently with cytochrome P450 inhibitors (cimetidine, macrolide antibiotics, antifungals) (Twycross et al.). Rifampicin inhibits reuptake of bile acids, and cholestyramine promotes sequestration of bile acids, thus both are useful for pruritus associated with cholestasis (Twycross et al.).

Psychosocial Care

The diagnosis of GI cancer invokes serious considerations regarding the quantity and quality of life. Patients may feel vulnerable and struggle with fears of isolation, discomfort, and uncertainty about the diagnosis and treatment. They may experience a variety of psychological states, such as denial, anxiety, and depression.

In a theory of cognitive adaptation, Taylor (1983) indicated that people experiencing actual or perceived life-threatening events such as cancer attempt to maintain or improve their sense of quality of life through cognitive restructuring processes, such as constructing meaning from the experience and restoration of control and self-esteem. Coward (1997) outlined diagnosis, completion of active treatment, and progression of disease as three pivotal points in the cancer trajectory. During this time, oncology nurses are positioned to assist patients and their families with clarification of values and personal choices and in establishing connections of similarity in order to construct meaning and find purpose.

At the point of diagnosis, patients and families may experience feelings of fear, shock, disbelief, aloneness, isolation, and loss of control. They often reach out for support and information about the diagnosis and treatment. They seek to restore control by assigning a cause to the diagnosis as a means for preventive action in personal recurrence or educating others for primary prevention. During this time, interventions include active listening and assisting the patient and family with referrals and resources that offer informational and emotional support. Patients and families should be encouraged to share experiences and establish connections that offer opportunities for new resources and support (Coward, 1997).

When active treatment is complete, issues of survivorship arise for the patient and family. Uncertainty exists about the future and the ability to manage the physical, social, and emotional long-term effects from treatment, with only interim follow-up visits with the healthcare team. Interventions at this time include physical assessments and addressing concerns for changes in relationships, body image, and role functions.

Referrals to professionally facilitated peer support groups are helpful for addressing concerns, making connections with other survivors, and promoting adjustment and restoring control (Coward, 1997).

Disease progression is the third pivotal point on the cancer trajectory. At this time, hopes and dreams are articulated and should be assessed for their impact on treatment decisions. Interventions should include encouragement of discussions about hopes and aspirations and assisting with identification of the most valued things in life. This will help in identifying and using available resources that may help to reduce gaps between expectations and reality (Coward, 1997).

Overall, psychosocial care for GI cancer diagnoses should include initial assessment for individual and family coping styles and available support systems and focus on disease process. Encourage the patient and family to actively participate in treatment decisions. Provide emotional, physical, and pharmaceutical support as indicated. Consider referral to additional support systems outside the family, such as recovering/survivor liaisons. Other supportive care treatments such as massage, relaxation, and guided imagery also may help in reduction of anxiety and an improved sense of control (Groen, 1999; Sauter & Coleman, 1999).

Palliative Care

Historically, palliative care was associated with end-of-life care and hospice. Today, palliative care can be viewed as a comprehensive, multidisciplinary approach to healthcare delivery that addresses the interpersonal, physical, psychological, social, and spiritual dimensions of care for patients and their families, with a primary objective of promoting well-being and enhancing the quality and meaning of life and death (Pickett, Cooley, & Gordon, 1998). In the physical dimension, well-being is evaluated and treated for alterations in appetite, sleep, bowel habits, nausea, strength, fatigue, and activities of daily living. In the spiritual dimension, religiosity, hope, uncertainty, positive changes, sense of purpose, suffering, meaning of pain, and transcendence are addressed. The psychological dimension addresses concentration, coping mechanisms, fear, anxiety, depression, sense of personal control and usefulness, and perceived happiness. The interpersonal and social dimensions address roles, relationships, support, and distress of family and friends, employment/financial concerns, isolation, appearance, affection, and sexuality (Pickett et al.). Palliative care encompasses all phases of the cancer illness trajectory, from diagnosis and treatment, follow-up/survivorship, recurrence or progression, to terminal disease and dying (Pasacreta & Pickett, 1998; Pickett et al.).

Palliative care for the patient with GI cancer often is in the setting of metastatic disease because of nonspecific symptoms that are present long before diagnosis. Chemotherapy, radiation therapy, or supportive care measures are used alone or in combination (Quinn & Reedy, 1999). Palliative care during this time focuses on increasing survival time and evaluating how physical symptoms affect other dimensions of care and overall quality of life. Major care tasks include making the patient comfortable through alleviation of physical symptoms, nutritional support, and pain control (Pickett et al., 1998; Quinn & Reedy). Chemotherapy is used to help control systemic disease, whereas radiation therapy is used for local control of tumor growth or to palliate symptoms that are secondary to tumor invasion, such as pain or dysphagia. Supportive care focuses on pain control, as well as nutritional and emotional support. When hospice care is introduced, it is important to help the patient and family to maintain dignity and as much control as possible and that the patient be kept comfortable (Quinn & Reedy).

Pain

Patients with cancer often experience pain, and both the patient and family fear this symptom. It has a direct impact on the patient's quality of life and often can be difficult to manage. Three types of pain are associated with patients with cancer: pain associated with the tumor, pain related to procedures and treatment, and pain unrelated to the cancer (McCaffery & Pasero, 1999). The exact mechanism of cancer pain is not known, and research continues into the pathophysiology of cancer pain. The patient with GI cancer may experience acute pain, chronic pain, or a combination. In acute pain, prostaglandins, serotonin, bradykinin, substance P, and histamine are released, stimulating sensory nerve endings. The neurons are excited and transmit a pain message to the peripheral nervous system and spinal cord. In chronic pain, the pain persists after the stimulus has diminished. Research is ongoing to determine the exact mechanism that causes pain to continue after the initial cause is removed (Paice, 2003).

Assessment of Pain

A comprehensive physical assessment should be performed on patients experiencing pain. Special focus should be placed on a neurologic assessment, including the cranial nerves. Sites of pain also need to be observed for signs of infection and skin breakdown and should be palpated and percussed to determine if there is tenderness (Paice, 2003).

When assessing pain, evaluate the onset, intensity, quality, aggravating and alleviating factors, and cultural considerations. Simple tools that are easy to understand, such as a 0–10 scale, should be used to quantify intensity. The Wong-Baker faces scale can be used in pediatrics or for patients who are unable to comprehend a 0–10 scale. When assessing pain quality, differentiate between nociceptive and neuropathic pain. Nociceptive pain generally relates to tissue damage. The two subtypes of nociceptive pain are somatic and visceral. Somatic pain is caused by damage to the musculoskeletal, cutaneous,

or deep tissues. Common types of somatic pain are bone pain and postsurgical pain. Descriptors often used by patients for this type of pain are sharp, throbbing, aching, or pressure-like. Visceral pain originates from damage or stretching of the abdominal or thoracic viscera. Patients often describe it as cramping, gnawing, or deep aching. It is rarely localized and can be referred from other sites. This is common in patients with GI cancers and often is seen in the pain syndromes associated with colon, rectal, and pancreatic cancers (McCaffery & Pasero, 1999; Paice, 2003). Neuropathic pain is another type of pain that is seen in patients with GI cancers. It often is described as burning, shooting, or "pins and needles." This pain is caused by central nervous system damage and can be caused by chemotherapeutic agents such as paclitaxel and cisplatin (McCaffery & Pasero).

Treatment of Cancer Pain

Treatment of cancer pain is quite complex, and guidelines are available to guide interventions. Nonpharmacologic treatment includes repositioning, guided imagery, therapeutic touch, relaxation techniques, yoga, and deep breathing. Oncology nurses can incorporate all of these interventions into the treatment of cancer-related pain, and they tend to work best when incorporated into a regimen combined with pharmacologic therapy (Paice, 2003).

The World Health Organization (WHO) and the National Comprehensive Cancer Network (NCCN) both provide useful evidence-based guidelines for the treatment of cancer-related pain. WHO uses a three-step analgesic ladder, which incorporates nonopioids, opioids, and adjuvant drugs to treat pain. Each step of the ladder addresses different intensities of pain and focuses on selecting analgesics on the basis of intensity. The first step suggests interventions using nonopioids, including a nonsteroidal anti-inflammatory drug or acetaminophen. If pain is not relieved with a nonopioid, the ladder suggests adding an opioid. Each level builds on the previous level of the ladder and does not recommend discontinuing the medication initiated on the previous step. Step three incorporates using an opioid that is appropriate for severe pain with or without adjuvant pain medicine. For example, someone on step three of the WHO ladder should be receiving a drug similar to oxycodone; acetaminophen with codeine would not be appropriate (McCaffery & Pasero, 1999). As discussed in the constipation section, begin a bowel regimen as soon as a patient is placed on opioid therapy.

NCCN guidelines for the treatment of cancer pain are similar in nature to the WHO guidelines but are more comprehensive and include guidelines on assessment of cancer pain. The NCCN guidelines also have three categories in treating pain, but they are separated into pain intensity ratings: 1–3, 4–6, and 7–10. The recommendations for treatment with medications are almost the same as the WHO guidelines, but NCCN also includes bowel regimens and psychosocial support. These guidelines also specifically address adjuvant therapy for pain, including nerve blocks, spinal opioids, and neuroaxial analgesia (NCCN, 2004). Additional useful resources for the treatment of pain can be found online (see Figure 7-2).

Figure 7-2. Useful Resources in Pain Management

- American Cancer Society: www.cancer.org
- American Pain Foundation: www.painfoundation.org
- American Society of Pain Management Nurses: www.aspmn.org
- City of Hope Pain Resource Center: http://cityofhope.org/prc/
- National Comprehensive Cancer Network: www.nccn.org
- Oncology Nursing Society: www.ons.org
- Partners for Understanding Pain: www.understandingpain.org
- World Health Organization: www.who.int/cancer/palliative /painladder/en/

Summary

Patients with GI cancers can experience a great number of debilitating symptoms and look to the oncology nurse for relief. By staying abreast of the nursing and medical literature on topics such as effective interventions for pain, diarrhea, mucositis, and skin changes, the nurse can greatly alleviate, or even prevent, these significant factors that affect quality of life.

References

Anthony, L. (2003). New strategies for the prevention and reduction of cancer treatment-induced diarrhea. *Seminars in Oncology Nursing, 19*(4 Suppl. 3), 17–21.

Arce, D.A., Ermocilla, C.A., & Costa, H. (2002). Evaluation of constipation. *American Family Physician, 65,* 2283–2290.

Avila, J.G. (2004). Pharmacologic treatment of constipation in cancer patients. *Cancer Control, 11*(Suppl. 3), 11–18.

Avritscher, E.B., Cooksley, C.D., & Elting, L.S. (2004). Scope and epidemiology of cancer therapy induced oral and gastrointestinal mucositis. *Seminars in Oncology Nursing, 20,* 3–10.

Brown, C.G., & Wingard, J. (2004). Clinical consequences of oral mucositis. *Seminars in Oncology Nursing, 20*(1), 16–21.

Childress, J., & Lokich, J. (2003). Cutaneous hand and foot toxicity associated with cancer chemotherapy. *American Journal of Clinical Oncology, 26,* 435–436.

Cope, D. (2001). Management of chemotherapy-induced diarrhea and constipation. *Nursing Clinics of North America, 36,* 695–707.

Coward, D. (1997). Constructing meaning from the experience of cancer. *Seminars in Oncology Nursing, 13,* 248–251.

Cunningham, R. (2004). The anorexia-cachexia syndrome. In C.H. Yarbro, M.H. Frogge, & M. Goodman (Eds.), *Cancer symptom management* (3rd ed., pp. 135–155). Sudbury, MA: Jones and Bartlett.

Cunningham, R.S., & Bell, R. (2000). Nutrition in cancer: An overview. *Seminars in Oncology Nursing, 16,* 90–98.

Curtas, S. (1999). Diagnosing gastrointestinal malignancies. *Seminars in Oncology Nursing, 15,* 10–16.

Davis, M.P., Frandsen, J.L., Walsh, D., Andresen, S., & Taylor, S. (2003). Mirtazapine for pruritus. *Journal of Pain and Symptom Management, 25,* 288–291.

Drossman, D.A. (2001). *Rome II: Functional gastrointestinal disorders.* Lawrence, KS: Allen Press.

Dunphy, R.C., & Verne, G.N. (2001). Drug treatment options for irritable bowel syndrome: Managing for success. *Drugs and Aging, 18,* 201–211.

Engelking, C. (2003). Diarrhea. In C.H. Yarbro, M.H. Frogge, & M. Goodman (Eds.), *Cancer symptom management* (3rd ed., pp. 528–558). Sudbury, MA: Jones and Bartlett.

Epstein, J., & Schubert, M. (2004). Managing pain in mucositis. *Seminars in Oncology Nursing, 20,* 30–37.

Epstein, J.B., Truelove, E.L., Oien, H., Allison, C., Le, N.D., & Epstein, M.S. (2001). Oral topical doxepin rinse; analgesic effect in patients with oral mucosal pain due to cancer therapy. *Oral Oncology, 37,* 632–637.

Etter, L., & Myers, S.A. (2002). Pruritus in systemic disease: Mechanisms and management. *Dermatologic Clinics, 20,* 459–472.

Farooqi, S., Bevan, J.S., Sheppard, M.C., & Wass, J.A. (1999). The therapeutic value of somatostatin and its analogues. *Pituitary, 3,* 79–88.

Gallagher, J. (1995). Management of cutaneous symptoms. *Seminars in Oncology Nursing, 11,* 239–247.

Gerbrecht, B.M. (2003). Current Canadian experience with capecitabine: Partnering with patients to optimize therapy. *Cancer Nursing, 26,* 161–167.

Glaser, E., & Grogan, L. (1999). Molecular genetics of gastrointestinal malignancies. *Seminars in Oncology Nursing, 15,* 3–9.

Grant, E. (Ed.). (1999). Use of sucralfate enemas for radiation proctitis. *Druginform, 20*(5), 29–31.

Grant, M., & Kravits, K. (2000). Symptoms and their impact on nutrition. *Seminars in Oncology Nursing, 16,* 113–121.

Grant, M., & Ropka, M. (1996). Alterations in nutrition. In R. McCorkle, M. Grant, M. Frank-Stromborg, & S. Baird (Eds.), *Cancer nursing: A comprehensive textbook* (2nd ed., pp. 919–943). Philadelphia: Saunders.

Groen, K. (1999). Primary and metastatic liver cancer. *Seminars in Oncology Nursing, 15,* 48–57.

Inui, A. (1999). Cancer anorexia-cachexia syndrome: Are neuropeptides the key? *Cancer Research, 59,* 4493–4501.

Inui, A. (2002). Cancer anorexia-cachexia syndrome: Current issues in research and management. *CA: A Cancer Journal for Clinicians, 52,* 72–91.

Keefe, D., Gibson, R., & Hauer-Jensen, M. (2004). Gastrointestinal mucositis. *Seminars in Oncology Nursing, 20,* 38–47.

Koppel, R.A., & Boh, E.E. (2001). Cutaneous reaction to chemotherapeutic agents. *American Journal of the Medical Sciences, 321,* 327–335.

Lamers, C.B., Bijlstra, A.M., & Harris, A.G. (1993). Octreotide, a long acting somatostatin analog in the management of postoperative dumping syndrome. An update. *Digestive Diseases and Sciences, 38,* 359–364.

Lidstone, V., & Thorns, A. (2001). Pruritus in cancer patients. *Cancer Treatment Reviews, 27,* 305–312.

McCaffery, M., & Pasero, C. (1999). *Pain: Clinical manual* (2nd ed.). St. Louis, MO: Mosby.

McGuire, M. (2000). Nutritional care of surgical oncology patients. *Seminars in Oncology Nursing, 16,* 128–134.

McMillan, S. (2002). Presence and severity of constipation in hospice patients with advanced cancer. *American Journal of Hospice and Palliative Care, 19,* 426–430.

Miaskowski, C. (1996). Oncologic emergencies. In R. McCorkle, M. Grant, M. Frank-Stromborg, & S. Baird (Eds.), *Cancer nursing: A comprehensive textbook* (2nd ed., pp. 919–943). Philadelphia: Saunders.

Nagore, E., Insa, A., & Sanmartin, O. (2000). Antineoplastic therapy-induced palmar plantar erythrodysesthesia ('hand-foot') syndrome. Incidence, recognition and management. *American Journal of Clinical Dermatology, 1*(4), 225–234.

National Cancer Institute Cancer Therapy Evaluation Program. (2003). *Common terminology criteria for adverse events, version 3.0.* Retrieved May 11, 2006, from http://ctep.cancer.gov/forms/CTCAEv3.pdf

National Comprehensive Cancer Network. (2004). *NCCN clinical practice guidelines in oncology, version 2.2004.* Jenkintown, PA: Author.

Nettina, S.M. (2001). *Lippincott manual of nursing practice* (7th ed.). Boston: Lippincott Williams & Wilkins.

O'Connor, K. (1999). Gastric cancer. *Seminars in Oncology Nursing, 15,* 26–35.

Paice, J.A. (2003). Pain. In C.H. Yarbro, M.H. Frogge, & M. Goodman (Eds.), *Cancer symptom management* (3rd ed., pp. 77–96). Sudbury, MA: Jones and Bartlett.

Pasacreta, J.V., & Pickett, M. (1998). Psychosocial aspects of palliative care. *Seminars in Oncology Nursing, 14,* 110–120.

Pascual Lopez, A., Rogue, I., Figuls, M., Urrutia Cuchi, G., Berenstein, E., Almenar Pasies, B., et al. (2004). Systematic review of megestrol acetate in the treatment of anorexia-cachexia syndrome. *Journal of Pain and Symptom Management, 27,* 360–369.

Peterson, D., Beck, S., & Keefe, D. (2004). Novel therapies. *Seminars in Oncology Nursing, 20,* 53–58.

Pickett, M., Cooley, M.E., & Gordon, D.B. (1998). Palliative care: Past, present, and future perspectives. *Seminars in Oncology Nursing, 14,* 86–94.

Piguet, V., & Borradori, L. (2002). Pyogenic granuloma-like lesions during capecitabine therapy. *British Journal of Dermatology, 147,* 1270–1272.

Quinn, K., & Reedy, A. (1999). Esophageal cancer: Therapeutic approaches and nursing care. *Seminars in Oncology Nursing, 15,* 17–25.

Rothenberg, M.L., Meropol, N.J., Poplin, E., Van Cutsem, E., & Wadler, S. (2001). Mortality associated with irinotecan plus bolus fluorouracil/leucovorin: Summary findings of an independent panel. *Journal of Clinical Oncology, 19,* 3801–3806.

Rutledge, D., & Engelking, C. (1998). Cancer-related diarrhea: Selected findings of a national survey of oncology nurse experiences. *Oncology Nursing Forum, 25,* 861–872.

Saddler, D., & Ellis, C. (1999). Colorectal cancer. *Seminars in Oncology Nursing, 15,* 58–69.

Sauter, P., & Coleman, J. (1999). Pancreatic cancer: A continuum of care. *Seminars in Oncology Nursing, 15,* 36–47.

Scheithauer, W., & Blum, J. (2004). Coming to grips with hand-foot syndrome. Insights from clinical trials evaluating capecitabine. *Oncology(Williston Park), 18,* 1161–1168, 1173.

Smith, S. (2001). Evidence-based management of constipation in the oncology patient. *European Journal of Oncology Nursing, 5,* 18–25.

Sonis, S. (2004). Pathobiology of mucositis. *Seminars in Oncology Nursing, 20,* 11–15.

Stepp, L., & Pakiz, T.S. (2001). Anorexia and cachexia in advanced cancer. *Nursing Clinics of North America, 36,* 735–744.

Stern, J., & Ippoliti, J. (2003). Management of acute cancer treatment-induced diarrhea. *Seminars in Oncology Nursing, 19*(4 Suppl. 3), 11–16.

Taylor, S. (1983). Adjustment to life threatening events: A theory of cognitive adaptation. *American Psychologist, 38,* 1161–1173.

Twycross, R., Greaves, M.W., Handwerker, H., Jones, E.A., Libretto, S.E., Szepietowski, J.C., et al. (2003). Itch: Scratching more than the surface. *Quarterly Journal of Medicine, 96*(1), 7–26.

Viele, C. (2003). Overview of chemotherapy-induced diarrhea. *Seminars in Oncology Nursing, 19*(4 Suppl. 3), 2–5.

Wong, P.W., & Kadakia, S. (1999). How to deal with chronic constipation. *Postgraduate Medicine, 106*(6), 199–200, 203–204, 207–210.

Yarbro, C., & Seiz, A. (2004). Pruritis. In C.H. Yarbro, M.H. Frogge, & M. Goodman (Eds.), *Cancer symptom management* (3rd ed., pp. 97–110). Sudbury, MA: Jones and Bartlett.

Zylicz, Z., Krajnik, M., Sorge, A.A., & Costantini, M. (2003). Paroxetine in the treatment of severe non-dermatological pruritus: A randomized, controlled trial. *Journal of Pain and Symptom Management, 26,* 1105–1112.

CHAPTER 8

Evidence-Based Practice: Where We Are Now

Joyce P. Griffin-Sobel, RN, PhD, AOCN®, APRN,BC

Evidence-Based Practice Defined

Evidence-based practice (EBP) is a systematic approach to using the best evidence available to guide clinical care. Sackett (2000) defined it as "integrating individual clinical expertise with the best available external evidence from systematic research" (p. 7). It is a vehicle for assessing knowledge for its appropriate use in practice. Projects to maximize the applicability of research data for practice have taken many forms over the years. In nursing, research utilization projects such as the Western Interstate Commission for Higher Education (WICHE) project and the Conduct and Utilize Research in Nursing (CURN) project were multiyear programs that developed practice protocols, such as the prevention of decubiti, based on research data (Burns & Grove, 2005). EBP involves defining a problem and generating a specific clinical question; searching for, finding, and evaluating evidence; planning an intervention that uses the evidence in a practice situation; and evaluating the results (Sackett). The process of EBP began in medicine and now is an expectation of healthcare practice by patients, government agencies, payors, accrediting bodies, and other professionals (Pravikoff, Tanner, & Pierce, 2005). The problem is that many healthcare professionals do not know how to find the information they need or how to utilize it if they find it. An alarming study by Pravikoff et al. surveyed 760 nurses with national geographic distribution; 48% had a bachelor's degree or higher, and 60% worked in a hospital. Sixty-one percent of the nurses needed information for clinical care at least once a week, but most (67%) sought that information from a colleague and seldom utilized journals or hospital libraries. Fewer than half of the nurses had knowledge of the term "evidence-based practice," 82% had never used the hospital library, and 77% had not received instruction in the use of electronic databases and resources. Nurses ranked the primary barriers to EBP as a lack of value for research in practice, lack of understanding of databases, and difficulty accessing research materials. The authors concluded that nurses in the United States are not ready for EBP because they do not value research, lack information literacy skills, and have limited access to good information. This sobering study highlights the importance of instilling the value of research, lifelong learning, and information literacy skills into basic nursing education programs.

One essential resource to ensure that nursing practice is based on evidence is point-of-care databases. Resources such as PDA tools with guidelines and care maps, training in health information literacy with access to medical librarians, easy-to-use databases, and electronic journals are all key components to encourage nurses to base care on sound evidence. Multiple models are available to guide the process of EBP for nurses. The Stetler Model of Research Utilization to Facilitate Evidence-Based Practice (Stetler, 2001) and the Iowa Model of Evidence-Based Practice to Promote Quality Care (Titler et al., 2001) are two widely used models. The Oncology Nursing Society (ONS) also has developed a collection of resources for developing skill in the process of EBP. The process is defined as problem identification, finding evidence, critique of the evidence, summarizing evidence, application to practice, and evaluation (ONS, 2005). Each step has a Web page with numerous links for references and further information (see Figures 8-1 and 8-2).

Although it is beyond the scope of this book to discuss the process of EBP in depth, nurses should understand the hierarchy of evidence. Although different schema exist, the majority regard systematic reviews or meta-analysis of randomized clinical trials as the highest level of evidence (level I), followed, in decreasing order, by evidence from a single randomized controlled trial, evidence from controlled trials without randomization, evidence from case-control studies, evidence from systematic reviews of descriptive studies, and evidence from expert committees (Guyatt & Rennie, 2002). Very few nursing studies are in the categories of highest levels of evidence.

Figure 8-1. Problem Identification

A problem is the statement of a question that needs to be answered or a situation that needs a solution. The problem emerges from a clinical situation in which there is a knowledge gap or uncertainty regarding the "best" response to the situation.
- Recognize that a problem exists.
- Phrase the problem accurately to facilitate the search for a precise answer.

Developing the question
This is a crucial step in the evidence-based practice (EBP) process; therefore, the right people must be involved in this process, and adequate time must be allotted.

Team members
- Design a multidisciplinary team to work on the entire EBP process.
- The group should represent all of the key healthcare providers for the particular clinical situation in question; for example, one group may have representatives from medicine, nursing, pharmacy, physical therapy, nutritional support, case management, and home care. Some level of administration also is helpful to have represented on the team.
- Representation on the team often facilitates support for the recommended practice change that is the outcome of the EBP process.
- Co-leaders are accepted more readily. Ideal co-leaders for many groups may be an advanced practice nurse and a physician.

Time
- Adequate time must be allotted for this phase in the EBP process.
- Adequate time is needed to consider and develop the best question. The more exact the question, the more focused the search for evidence can be.
- Prioritize by asking, "What is the most important issue for this current situation?" or "What issue should be addressed first?"

Essential components of a question
A question should contain the following essential components to guide the search for evidence:
- Patient or situation being addressed
- Phenomenon being considered
- Comparison intervention, when relevant
- Clinical outcomes of interest.

Knowledge gaps
Problems may identify knowledge gaps within a clinical situation in the following areas.
- Diagnosis: Questions regarding the selection and interpretation of diagnostic tests
- Prognosis: Questions regarding the likely patient's clinical outcome
- Therapy: Questions regarding the selection of treatments that are most beneficial
- Prevention: Questions regarding screening and prevention methods to reduce the risk of disease
- Education: Questions regarding best teaching strategies for colleagues, patients, or family members

Note. From "Evidence-Based Practice Resource Area—Problem Identification," by the Oncology Nursing Society, 2005. Retrieved July 18, 2006, from http://onsopcontent.ons.org/toolkits/evidence/Process/problem.shtml. Copyright 2005 by the Oncology Nursing Society. Adapted with permission.

Nursing Research Literature in Gastrointestinal Cancers

Before one can use evidence in nursing practice, a substantial body of research must exist upon which to draw. To summarize research on gastrointestinal (GI) cancers and their management by nurses, the author conducted a literature search in 2006. Databases utilized were MEDLINE®, CINAHL®, the Virginia Henderson Library of Sigma Theta Tau, and Cochrane Library Reviews. Search terms used were neoplasms of the colon, rectum, anus, stomach, and esophagus; nursing; and research. Set criteria were year (1990–2006), language (English), and peer-reviewed publications. More than 11,700 articles were published about colon cancers, with close to 4,000 of those written in the last five years. Stomach cancer had 12,400 articles listed in the MEDLINE database, and 9,100 were listed for

rectal cancer. The majority of these articles were descriptions of pharmacologic trials and medical management, clinical reviews, or descriptions of surgical techniques.

In the nursing databases, far fewer publications were noted, with 458 articles written on colon cancer between 2000 and 2006. Negligible numbers were found in the nursing literature on other types of GI cancers. The vast majority of these publications were clinical articles describing disease, medical management, symptom management, and psychosocial interventions. Papers describing studies conducted by nurses fell into two primary categories: screening behaviors and psychosocial care, which included communication. These research studies were published in a variety of journals, including *Journal of Nursing Scholarship, Nursing Research, Clinical Journal of Oncology Nursing, Cancer Nursing, Oncology Nursing Forum, Psy-*

Figure 8-2. Finding the Evidence

The evidence needed in an evidence-based practice (EBP) effort may be found in a variety of sources, from computerized bibliographical databases to your own quality improvement department. In trying to find evidence, nurses are urged to get help. For one reason, finding evidence is very time consuming even when done with maximum efficiency and more people. And second, those familiar with a method may search and find better sources of information.

A systematic approach to finding evidence
- Have a clearly defined topic.
- Review all existing hospital/agency policies/procedures for current practice standards.
- Determine if the recommended practice is being implemented. Quality improvement (QI) data may give you this information or a QI project may be needed.
- Check for external standards/policies on the topic.
- Find any systematic or integrative reviews on the topic or meta-analyses.
- Search for primary research literature using a computerized bibliographic database.

Principles of searching computerized bibliographic databases
- Plan your search and break your topic into pieces. Example: patient education in ovarian cancer patients may be searched by
  1) Seeking literature about patient education
  2) Seeking literature about ovarian cancer and then having the database list any articles that are in both search results. You can limit your search by information about patients (e.g., gender, age, ethnicity) or type of publication (e.g., clinical, research, instrument).

Successful searches
- Find information about one or more articles that seem pertinent to your EBP project.
- Seek the full text version of each pertinent article and proceed to appraising the findings.

Unsuccessful searches
- Go through this process several times; you may need to get assistance.
- Questions to ask if search is not successful: Using the correct terms to search? Using the most appropriate databases or sites?
- Be aware that some topics have little published research and therefore will lead you to an "unsuccessful" search.

Note. From "Evidence-Based Practice Resource Area—Finding the Evidence," by the Oncology Nursing Society, 2005. Retrieved July 18, 2006, from http://onsopcontent.ons.org/toolkits/evidence/Process/evidence.shtml. Copyright 2005 by the Oncology Nursing Society. Adapted with permission.

---

cho-Oncology, and *Health Education Research.* In addition to research studies specifically addressing GI cancer care, research studies exist within the specialty areas of wound, ostomy, and continence; pain management; and gastroenterology nursing that provide guidance on caring for patients with ostomies, fecal and urinary incontinence, obstructing lesions, pain, and disorders of elimination. Those studies will not be reviewed here but are a valuable resource to the oncology nurse caring for patients with GI cancers.

Screening Behaviors

Colorectal cancer (CRC) is preventable with appropriate screening. The literature shows that being screened for CRC is not high on the priority list of many people. Whether it be fecal occult blood testings, sigmoidoscopy, or colonoscopy, studies have shown that the public receives inconsistent recommendations about CRC screening from their healthcare providers, were concerned about the efficacy of the test, and were embarrassed and afraid over the possibility of a cancer being found (Rawl, Menon, Champion, Foster, & Skinner, 2000). Many individuals studied had not even thought about

being screened, even when they had a first-degree relative with a diagnosis of colon cancer (Rawl et al., 2005). These findings were confirmed elsewhere (Jacobs, 2002). Barriers to being screened included having no symptoms, lack of physician recommendations, cost, and lack of knowledge about the tests (Rawl et al., 2000, 2005). In some patients, a fatalism about cancer influenced cancer screening behaviors, and this fatalism was highest in older African American women (Powe & Finnie, 2003). Cancer fatalism is defined as the belief that death is inevitable when cancer is present, and this was the only statistically significant predictor of CRC screening (Powe, 1995; Powe & Finnie). Researchers studied an intervention directed at reducing cancer fatalism (Powe & Weinrich, 1999). A video with content on CRC, cancer fatalism, spirituality, and hope was tested on rural older adults (N = 70). The group that witnessed the video had a significantly greater decrease in cancer fatalism scores and a greater increase in CRC knowledge than the control group.

Another study found that knowledge about CRC and screening in a predominantly African American sample was low, and these patients were unlikely to participate in a screening activity compared to Caucasians (Powe, Finnie, &

Ko, 2006). Younger patients were no more knowledgeable than older adults in this study. These results were verified in another study (Green & Kelly, 2004). In a sample of African American men and women older than 50 (N = 100), less than half had a passing knowledge of CRC as a disease or screening recommendations. The majority of subjects expressed embarrassment about screening and concern about potential pain with screening tests. Barriers to screening that were identified were fear of discovering cancer and not knowing how to schedule a screening test. Another study found that older women who were caring for their spouse also underutilized cancer screening for CRC, despite the fact that older adults are at higher risk for CRC (Sarna & Chang, 2000). Using qualitative methods, one study revealed 10 themes influencing decisions about participating in colorectal screening, including competing demands on their time, preparation for the procedure, the discomfort of the test, fear of cancer, no symptoms, negative experiences of others, and the negative image of aging (Wackerbath, Peters, & Haist, 2005). Much education must be undertaken to inform individuals about the value of screening, and the medium for that education also must be evaluated.

Psychosocial Concerns

Studies included both quantitative and qualitative methodologies. Northouse, Schafer, Tipton, and Metivier (1999) interviewed patients with colon cancer and their spouses to determine their concerns about the diagnosis. An additional aim was to identify ways nurses could assist patients and spouses to cope with treatment. Results showed that spouses tended to be more negatively affected by the cancer diagnosis than were patients, with most reporting lifestyle and role changes. Patients reported more functional changes. Subjects reported a need for more information about treatments and management of symptoms.

In interviews with 14 newly diagnosed patients with stage III or IV colorectal cancer, patients described distressing interactions with physicians and feelings of disrupted lives, losses, being unprepared, and rethinking parenting. Other significant areas of concern were trying to cope with the diagnosis by staying positive and assessing meaning from the diagnosis (Houldin & Lewis, 2006).

Klemm, Miller, and Fernsler (2000) studied the demands of illness in patients with CRC and found considerable distress in the personal meaning domain, with the majority of patients reporting concern about the value of life or how long they may live. Younger patients had higher demands of illness. Another study found that the demands of illness in people with CRC were higher in men, younger patients, and those with advanced disease (Fernsler, Klemm, & Miller, 1999). People who reported higher levels of spiritual well-being had significantly lower demands of illness related to physical symptoms and treatment issues, although the correlations were weak. Spiritual well-being was defined as the affirmation of life in relationship to a higher power, nurturing the concept of wholeness (Fernsler et al.).

Communication and the difficulties therein have been well described in the nursing literature, both from the patient's perspective and the provider's. Sheldon, Barrett, and Ellington (2006) interviewed nurses to explore perceptions of difficult communication within the nurse-patient relationship. Although not confined to the oncology patient, themes were applicable to patients with cancer. Nurses described specific diagnoses and clinical situations; patient and family emotions; the nurses' emotions and coping behaviors with difficult communication; and the nurse-physician-patient relationship. Nurses noted the lack of educational content on communication. A literature review (Sheldon, 2005) validated these findings and demonstrated the value of training programs in communication skills.

Other papers demonstrated that patients with cancer have unmet communication needs (Hack, Degner, & Parker, 2005), and patient-based interventions, such as prompt sheets, aid their communication with providers (Parker, Davison, Tishelman, & Brundage, 2005).

The ability of the patient to perform self-care has become increasingly important as hospitalization time has decreased. For a patient to learn self-care and follow instructions, he or she must have adequate health literacy or a "constellation of skills, including the ability to perform basic reading and numerical tasks required to function in the health care environment" (American Medical Association, 1999, p. 553). Low health literacy skills are associated with low rates of medical screening, and 90 million adults in the United States have inadequate reading skills (Agre, Stieglitz, & Milstein, 2006). Many healthcare providers do not know the literacy level of their patients, and patients with poor literacy skills often have inadequate knowledge to manage their disease and do not remember self-care instructions. Health literacy should be assessed in patients using a variety of available tools (Agre et al.) and alternative means of instruction, such as videos or audiotapes. Studies have not examined a variety of populations or the tailoring of specific media to those population characteristics.

In the area of telehealth, a project was undertaken to manage nursing care of patients with new ostomies (Bohnenkamp, McDonald, Lopez, Krupinski, & Blackett, 2004). Patients were managed with traditional home-health nursing care or by telenursing, defined for the study as using telecommunications and information technology to move the point of care to the home of the patient. Using phone calls and a monitor that hooked up to the TV, patients in the telenursing group were educated on ostomy care. The home-health group was visited at home in the traditional manner. The telenursing group reported more satisfaction with their care after discharge and were able to master the skills needed to perform self-care on a new stoma. This study exemplifies the creativity that is possible in meeting the needs of patients.

Directions for the Future

Research priorities in both oncology nursing and gastroenterology nursing have been identified. A recent study of nursing research priorities of oncology nurses identified the following topics as research priorities: acute and chronic pain, infection rates and control, job satisfaction, nurse-patient ratios and staffing, and nurse retention (Cohen, Harle, Woll, Despa, & Munsell, 2004). In 2000, ONS conducted a survey to prioritize research in oncology nursing (Ropka et al., 2002). The highest-ranking research priorities were pain, quality of life, early detection of cancer, prevention or risk education, neutropenia, or immunosuppression. In 2002, Griffin-Sobel and Suozzo examined research priorities of nurses caring for gastroenterology patients. Leading priorities were enhancing comfort in patients undergoing endoscopic procedures and determining optimum methods of sterilizing endoscopes for infection control.

Clinical research questions, such as those addressing alterations in pain, fatigue, infection, bowel function, and quality-of-life concerns, need to be studied in populations with GI cancer. Many nursing research questions on a multitude of symptoms have used patients with breast cancer for the sample, which severely limits the evidence base for the care of patients with other cancers.

Priority areas for the future should include prevention and early detection. Many GI cancers are preventable. Screening for CRC has been repeatedly demonstrated to be effective. Lifestyle alterations in diet, exercise, and avoidance of carcinogens such as tobacco have been well described in medical and epidemiologic literature in reducing the risk of cancers, and yet obesity, sedentary lifestyles, and smoking continue to be major public health problems. In the Nurses' Health Study, women with stages I–III colorectal cancer reduced their risk of mortality by increasing their physical activity, independent of prediagnosis levels of physical activity (Meyerhardt, Giovannucci, et al., 2006). For patients with stage III colon cancer, beyond surgical resection and chemotherapy, physical activity reduced the risk of cancer recurrence and mortality (Meyerhardt, Heseltine, et al., 2006). Only by linking research questions across disciplines can meaningful solutions be achieved. Behavioral theories, such as the Transtheoretical Model, have guided interventions in cancer prevention, with promising results in smoking cessation, dietary guidance, and obesity reduction (Gotay, 2005; Prochaska et al., 1994). This model would be very appropriate for nursing-sensitive studies. Likewise, effectively increasing participation in screening for early detection, particularly in populations with limited socioeconomic means or in those who possess cultural barriers to screening, is an area in great need of study. Nursing research has identified some of the barriers to screening, including fear and lack of symptomatology. Interventions aimed at educating the public about the disease and the efficacy of screening techniques would enhance the effectiveness of preventive tech-

niques. Specific populations need to be studied to ascertain which groups have cultural barriers to screening behaviors. Little is known about attitudes of Hispanics, Asians, Native Americans, and others toward preventive behaviors. Likewise, linking nursing research questions to those clinical trials examining various chemopreventive agents would expand the knowledge base in both disciplines. Studies examining dietary changes also are needed. The role of diet and alcohol in the etiology of esophageal, gastric, and colon cancers is well described, but behavioral change is difficult for most people. Studies are needed to examine the most effective methods to facilitate and maintain dietary changes.

The health disparities in incidence and death rates from cancer based on race, socioeconomic status, or geographic location have been well described previously. Health disparities in diagnosis, treatment, and survival from CRC exist among African Americans, Asian Americans, Pacific Islanders, Hispanics, and Native Americans. To address the myriad of research questions involved in this topic would involve professionals from medicine, nursing, public health, policy specialists, health economics, and the public. Cost and physicians' recommendations regarding screening are significant barriers to CRC screening. There is also a demonstrated lack of knowledge in minority populations about the risk factors for CRC and dietary and other preventive strategies. Education about diet and other preventive measures could be started at a younger age. Older patients, particularly African Americans, need more information about CRC to increase their knowledge of the disease and the importance of screening. Screening tests should be thoroughly described to eliminate the fear of pain. Educational interventions using a variety of media and sources could be studied to ascertain the most effective strategies for particular segments of the population. Although Internet-based information is an effective tool for some populations, it is not the preference of many African Americans (Powe et al., 2006). Determining tailored interventions to convey the importance of preventive and early detection measures is an essential component in reducing the disparities between races in CRC. Primary care providers, particularly those serving minority populations, need to be studied to determine the factors involved in inconsistent or nonexistent recommendations related to CRC screening.

Symptom management self-care would be the third area for research attention, particularly patient self-management techniques. Although knowledge is available for handling some GI-specific symptoms, such as diarrhea, nausea, and vomiting, other areas are in great need of study. Patient education and effective use of health literacy information is important to patient self-management in the home and community. One important study looked at the information needs of older adult patients discharged home after cancer surgery (Hughes, Hodgson, Muller, Robinson, & McCorkle, 2000). Patients expressed the need for more information on numerous topics, including course of illness, pain management, wound care, and community resources. What are the most effective ways that one can convey information to a patient to allow him or her to feel competent with self-care? Assessing health literacy rapidly is a difficult task, yet it is essential to individualizing patient education.

Lastly, survivorship is becoming an increasingly important issue for people cured of their cancers. During the summer of 2005, the *American Journal of Nursing (AJN)* organized an invitational symposium on cancer survivorship. Some of the participants were survivors, but most were nurses. The results of the conference, the State of the Science on Nursing Approaches to Managing Late and Long-Term Sequelae of Cancer and Cancer Treatment, were published as a supplement to *AJN* in March 2006, and the executive summary appeared in *AJN* (Houldin, Curtiss, & Haylock, 2006a) and in the *Clinical Journal of Oncology Nursing* (Houldin, Curtiss, & Haylock, 2006b).

More than 10 million cancer survivors exist in the United States, and many have long-standing health problems, such as metabolic syndrome, osteoporosis, thyroid problems, heart and lung problems, cataracts, and quality-of-life disruptions resulting from their therapy (Mitchell, 2006). CRC is becoming increasingly treatable and sometimes curable, and survivorship issues specific to GI cancers may emerge. Colon cancer treatment recently has expanded to include a host of new agents and combinations, and long-term issues from those agents may be of concern. One study found that survivors of CRC reported a heightened perception of risk, with frequent intrusive thoughts of anxiety and worry (Mullens, McCaul, Erickson, & Sandgren, 2004). Barriers to optimal care for cancer survivors included lack of knowledge on the part of healthcare professionals, cancer survivors, and the public; a lack of nursing research to inform the practice; and a lack of funding for survivor care. Strategies to overcome these barriers included publishing articles in medical and nursing journals, urging the inclusion of survivorship issues in nursing curricula, and including a survivorship component in current and new nursing studies and clinical trials. Patients need to be educated on survivorship issues, particularly coping with heightened anxiety. Studies are needed on the most effective methods of facilitating patient coping in transition to the survivor role.

Summary

Caring for patients with GI cancers is challenging and rewarding. Much of nurses' efforts have been directed at treating the effects of chemotherapy and surgery. Nursing studies need to build on that knowledge and explore interventions to prevent, alleviate, and treat the disease and its accompanying symptomatology. Educational strategies must be tailored to the specific needs of a particular population subset, and interdisciplinary research is important to comprehensively address research questions in a meaningful manner.

References

Agre, P., Stieglitz, E., & Milstein, G. (2006). The case for development of a new test of health literacy. *Oncology Nursing Forum, 33,* 283–289.

American Medical Association. (1999). Health literacy: Report of the Council on Scientific Affairs. *JAMA, 281,* 552–557.

Bohnenkamp, S., McDonald, P., Lopez, A., Krupinski, E., & Blackett, A. (2004). Traditional versus telenursing outpatient management of patients with cancer with new ostomies. *Oncology Nursing Forum, 31,* 1005–1010.

Burns, N., & Grove, S. (2005). *The practice of nursing research* (5th ed.). St. Louis, MO: Elsevier Saunders.

Cohen, M., Harle, M., Woll, A., Despa, S., & Munsell, M. (2004). Delphi survey of nursing research priorities. *Oncology Nursing Forum, 31,* 1011–1018.

Fernsler, J., Klemm, P., & Miller, M. (1999). Spiritual well-being and demands of illness in people with colorectal cancer. *Cancer Nursing, 22,* 134–140.

Gotay, C. (2005). Behavior and cancer prevention. *Journal of Clinical Oncology, 23,* 301–310.

Green, P., & Kelly, B. (2004). Colorectal cancer knowledge, perceptions, and behaviors in African Americans. *Cancer Nursing, 27,* 206–215.

Griffin-Sobel, J., & Suozzo, S. (2002). Nursing research priorities for the care of the client with a gastrointestinal disorder: A Delphi Survey. *Gastroenterology Nursing, 25*(5), 188–191.

Guyatt, G., & Rennie, D. (2002). *Users' guide to the medical literature.* Chicago: American Medical Association Press.

Hack, T., Degner, L., & Parker, P. (2005). The communication goals and needs of cancer patients: A review. *Psycho-Oncology, 14,* 831–845.

Houldin, A., Curtiss, C., & Haylock, P. (2006a). (Eds.). Executive summary: The state of the science on nursing approaches to managing late and long term sequelae of cancer and cancer treatment. *American Journal of Nursing, 106*(Suppl. 3), 54–59.

Houldin, A., Curtiss, C.P., & Haylock, P.J. (2006b). The state of the science on nursing approaches to managing late and long-term sequelae of cancer and cancer treatment. *Clinical Journal of Oncology Nursing, 10,* 327–332.

Houldin, A., & Lewis, F. (2006). Salvaging their normal lives: A qualitative study of patients with recently diagnosed advanced colorectal cancer. *Oncology Nursing Forum, 33,* 719–725.

Hughes, L., Hodgson, N., Muller, P., Robinson, L., & McCorkle, R. (2000). Information needs of elderly postsurgical cancer patients during the transition from hospital to home. *Journal of Nursing Scholarship, 32*(1), 25–30.

Jacobs, L. (2002). Health beliefs of first-degree relatives of individuals with colorectal cancer and participation in health maintenance visits: A population-based survey. *Cancer Nursing, 25,* 251–265.

Klemm, P., Miller, M., & Fernsler, J. (2000). Demands of illness in people treated for colorectal cancer. *Oncology Nursing Forum, 27,* 633–639.

Meyerhardt, J., Giovannucci, E., Holmes, M., Chan, A., Chan, J., Colditz, G., et al. (2006). Physical activity and survival after colorectal cancer diagnosis. *Journal of Clinical Oncology, 24,* 3527–3534.

Meyerhardt, J., Heseltine, D., Niedzwiecki, D., Hollis, D., Saltz, L., Mayer, R., et al. (2006). Impact of physical activity on cancer recurrence and survival in patients with stage III colon cancer: Findings from CALGB 89803. *Journal of Clinical Oncology, 24,* 3535–3541.

Mitchell, S.A. (2006). Cancer survivorship: An annotated bibliography. *American Journal of Nursing, 106*(Suppl. 3), e1–e19.

Retrieved October 6, 2006, from http://clinicalcenter.nih.gov /nursing/whoweare/mitc036d.pdf

Mullens, A., McCaul, K., Erickson, S., & Sandgren, A. (2004). Coping after cancer: Risk perceptions, worry and health behaviors among colorectal cancer survivors. *Psycho-Oncology, 13,* 367–376.

Northouse, L., Schafer, J., Tipton, J., & Metivier, L. (1999). The concerns of patients and spouses after a diagnosis of colon cancer. *Journal of Wound, Ostomy and Continence Nursing, 26*(1), 8–17.

Oncology Nursing Society. (2005). *Evidence-based practice resource area.* Retrieved July 18, 2006, from http://onsopcontent.ons. org/toolkits/evidence

Parker, P., Davison, B., Tishelman, C., & Brundage, M. (2005). What do we know about facilitating patient communication in the cancer care setting? *Psycho-Oncology, 14,* 848–858.

Powe, B. (1995). Fatalism among elderly African Americans: Effects on colorectal screening. *Cancer Nursing, 18,* 385–392.

Powe, B., & Finnie, R. (2003). Cancer fatalism: The state of the science. *Cancer Nursing, 26,* 454–465.

Powe, B., Finnie, R., & Ko, J. (2006). Enhancing knowledge of colorectal cancer among African Americans: Why are we waiting until age 50? *Gastroenterology Nursing, 29,* 42–49.

Powe, B., & Weinrich, S. (1999). An intervention to decrease cancer fatalism among rural elders. *Oncology Nursing Forum, 26,* 583–588.

Pravikoff, D., Tanner, A., & Pierce, S. (2005). Readiness of U.S. nurses for evidence-based practice. *American Journal of Nursing, 105*(9), 40–52.

Prochaska, J., Velicer, W., Rossi, J., Goldstein, M., Marcus, B., Rakowski, W., et al. (1994). Stages of change and decisional balance for 12 problem behaviors. *Health Psychology, 13,* 39–46.

Rawl, S., Menon, U., Champion, V., Foster, J., & Skinner, C. (2000). Colorectal cancer screening beliefs. *Cancer Practice, 8,* 32–37.

Rawl, S., Menon, U., Champion, V., May, F., Loehrer, P., Hunter, C., et al. (2005). Do benefits and barriers differ by stage of adoption for colorectal cancer screening? *Health Education Research, 20,* 137–148.

Ropka, M., Guterbock, T., Krebs, L., Murphy-Ende, K., Stetz, K., Summers, B., et al. (2002). Year 2000 Oncology Nursing Society research priorities survey. *Oncology Nursing Forum, 29,* 481–491.

Sackett, D. (2000). *Evidence-based medicine: How to practice and teach EBP.* London: Churchill-Livingstone.

Sarna, L., & Chang, B. (2000). Colon cancer screening among older women caregivers. *Cancer Nursing, 23,* 109–116.

Sheldon, L. (2005). Communication in oncology care: The effectiveness of skills training workshops for healthcare providers. *Clinical Journal of Oncology Nursing, 9,* 305–312.

Sheldon, L., Barrett, R., & Ellington, L. (2006). Difficult communication in nursing. *Journal of Nursing Scholarship, 38,* 141–147.

Stetler, C. (2001). Updating the Stetler Model of Research Utilization to facilitate evidence-based practice. *Nursing Outlook, 49,* 272–279.

Titler, M., Kleiber, C., Steelman, V., Rakel, B., Budreau, G., Everett, L., et al. (2001). The Iowa Model of Evidence-Based Practice to Promote Quality Care. *Critical Care Nursing Clinics of North America, 13,* 497–509.

Wackerbath, S., Peters, J., & Haist, S. (2005). Factors influencing colorectal cancer screening decisions. *Qualitative Health Research, 15,* 539–554.

Index

The letter f *following a page number indicates that relevant content appears in a figure; the letter* t, *in a table.*